Glycosylated Hemoglobins

CLINICAL AND BIOCHEMICAL ANALYSIS

A series of monographs and textbooks

EDITOR

Morton K. Schwartz

Chairman, Department of Biochemistry
Memorial Sloan-Kettering Cancer Center
New York, New York

1. Colorimetric and Fluorimetric Analysis of Organic Compounds and Drugs, *M. Pesez and J. Bartos*
2. Normal Values in Clinical Chemistry: Statistical Analysis of Laboratory Data, *Horace F. Martin, Benjamin J. Gudzinowicz, and Herbert Fanger*
3. Continuous Flow Analysis: Theory and Practice, *William B. Furman*
4. Handbook of Enzymatic Methods of Analysis, *George G. Guilbault*
5. Handbook of Radioimmunoassay, *edited by Guy E. Abraham*
6. The Hemoglobinopathies: Techniques of Identification, *Titus H. J. Huisman and J. H. P. Jonxis*
7. Automated Immunoanalysis (in two parts), *edited by Robert F. Ritchie*
8. Computers in the Clinical Laboratory: An Introduction, *E. Clifford Toren, Jr. and Arthur A. Eggert*
9. The Chromatography of Hemoglobin, *Walter A. Schroeder and Titus H. J. Huisman*
10. Nonisotopic Alternatives to Radioimmunoassay: Principles and Applications, *edited by Lawrence A. Kaplan and Amadeo J. Pesce*
11. Biochemical Markers for Cancer, *edited by T. Ming Chu*
12. Clinical and Biochemical Luminescence, *edited by Larry J. Kricka and Timothy J. N. Carter*
13. Advanced Interpretation of Clinical Laboratory Data, *edited by Camille Heusghem, Adelin Albert, and Ellis S. Benson*

14. Practical Immunoassay: The State of the Art, *edited by Wilfrid R. Butt*
15. Instrument Evaluation in Biomedical Sciences, *James L. Driscoll, Benjamin J. Gudzinowicz, and Horace F. Martin*
16. Chemi- and Bioluminescence, *edited by John G. Burr*
17. Ligand-Binder Assays: Labels and Analytical Strategies, *Larry J. Kricka*
18. Human Prenatal Diagnosis, *edited by Karen Filkins and Joseph F. Russo*
19. Glycosylated Hemoglobins: Methods of Analysis and Clinical Applications, *E. C. Abraham*

ADDITIONAL VOLUMES IN PREPARATION

Glycosylated Hemoglobins
Methods of Analysis and Clinical Applications

E. C. Abraham
Department of Cell and Molecular Biology
Medical College of Georgia
Augusta, Georgia

MARCEL DEKKER, INC. New York and Basel

Library of Congress Cataloging in Publication Data

Abraham, E. C.
Glycosylated hemoglobins.

(Clinical and biochemical analysis ; 19)
Includes bibliographies and indexes.
1. Glycosylated hemoglobin. 2. Glycosylated hemoglobin–Diagnostic use. 3. Hyperglycemia–Diagnosis. I. Title. II. Series. [DNLM: 1. Hemoglobin A, Glycosylated. 2. Hemoglobinopathies. W1 CL654 v.19 / WH 190 A159g]
QP99.3.G55A27 1985 612′.111 85-15913
ISBN 0-8247-7356-X

MARCEL DEKKER, INC.
270 Madison Avenue, New York, New York 10016

Current printing (last digit):
10 9 8 7 6 5 4 3 2 1

PRINTED IN THE UNITED STATES OF AMERICA

To Amminikutty, Jacob, Mini, and Jimmy

Preface

The nonenzymatic "browning" reaction, also called the Maillard reaction, was discovered during the early part of the twentieth century. Although the reaction was recognized in food in industry a long time ago, the importance of a similar process in biological systems became evident only after the discovery of the glycosylated hemoglobins and their increased presence in diabetic patients. Although nonenzymatic glycosylation of hemoglobin was originally thought to be rather specific for the β-chain amino terminus, it is now well established that several other sites are involved in this process. Now, we know that nonenzymatic glycosylation is not restricted to hemoglobin alone, because other proteins also undergo this posttranslational modification in tissues other than the red cell where the glucose transport is insulin independent. It may very well be that the secondary sequelae of diabetes can be considered as due to such postsynthetic protein modifications. Glycosylated hemoglobin may provide a conceptual framework to assess the pathogenesis of the secondary sequelae of diabetes. Two primary factors directly influencing the levels of glycosylated hemoglobins are (1) the glucose concentration dependence of nonenzymatic glycosylation, i.e., increased glycosylation with increased glucose concentration, and, therefore, relevance in diabetes, and (2) the time dependence of nonenzymatic glycosylation, i.e., increased or decreased levels of glycosylation depending upon the duration of the exposure of the hemoglobin molecule to glucose, and, therefore, relevance in hemolytic anemia.

This book is composed of a presentation of the structural and functional features of the various glycosylated hemoglobins, methods of their analyses, and the clinical applications of such analyses primarily in diabetes and secondarily in hemolytic anemias. It is directed to an audience of clinicians, clinical chemists, laboratory technologists, and research scientists. A brief description of the structural and functional aspects of the hemoglobin molecule in general is also presented, without which a discussion of the structure and function of glycosylated hemoglobins would not have been complete. The last chapter is devoted to a review of the work done in the glycosylation of proteins other than hemoglobin, which is a logical extension of the vast amount of information presented on hemoglobin glycosylation.

I am greatly indebted to several of my colleagues and collaborators, whose association has enabled me to make noteworthy contributions in hemoglobin glycosylation. They are Drs. T. H. J. Huisman, B. F. Cameron (Childrens Hospital, Cincinnati, Ohio), T. A. Huff, H. Ė. Fadel, M. M. Elseweidy, E. Bisse, and M. Volk (Isolab, Inc., Akron, Ohio); and Mrs. M. Stallings, Mrs. A. Abraham, Mrs. N. D. Cope, and Mr. R. E. Perry. Special thanks are due to Mrs. Ida O. Thomas for typing several versions of the manuscript and to Mrs. M. Stallings for numerous hours of library work.

I am immensely grateful to my mentors, namely, Dr. John F. Taylor (former Chairman, Department of Biochemistry, University of Louisville School of Medicine) and Dr. T. H. J. Huisman (Chairman, Department of Cell and Molecular Biology, Medical College of Georgia), who have introduced me to the vast area of hemoglobin research.

E. C. Abraham

Contents

Glycosylated Hemoglobins

1

Introduction and Historical Aspects

I. THE MAILLARD REACTION

The Maillard reaction was named after L. C. Maillard, who conducted pioneering work from 1912 to 1917 on sugar and amino acid condensation (1,2). The Maillard reaction is recognized in food industry as the "browning" reaction (3-5). The reaction scheme occurs in several stages. The first stage involves a condensation reaction between a free amino group and the carbonyl group of a reducing sugar such as glucose. The resulting product of the initial step is a reversible Schiff-base adduct and a molecule of water. Subsequent cyclization and isomerization (Amadori rearrangement) results in a 1-amino-1-deoxy-2-ketose. The complex polymerization reactions of the Amadori products yield both soluble and insoluble pigments in the final stage of the Maillard reaction. In the initial reaction both mono- and disaccharide reducing sugars can react with α-amino or ϵ-amino groups. The reactivity of these reducing sugars varies: aldopentoses are more reactive than aldohexoses, which in turn are more reactive than disaccharides. The quality and the properties of the food change following prolonged reaction of the proteins with carbohydrates.

Nonenzymatic browning can occur in dehydrated and semimoist foods during storage. This reaction in food products results from reducing compounds, primarily sugars, reacting with proteins, peptides, and amino acids, and leads to changes in the aesthetic, functional, and nutritional properties of the food in which the reaction occurs. Various physical factors (such as pH, water content, and the amount of the initial reactant species) can affect the Maillard reaction (3). High reactivity of the ϵ-amino group of the essential amino acid lysine with carbohydrates makes it chemically and nutritionally unavailable (4). For example, exposure of casein or soy protein to heat in the presence of glucose induces variable losses in lysine depending on the severity of the treatment (4).

II. NONENZYMATIC GLYCOSYLATION (GLYCATION)*

During the last decade, the biomedical sciences have become familiar with in vivo nonenzymatic glycosylation of proteins, hemoglobin in particular. The relationship of such glycosylation to diabetes mellitus has been the subject of extensive investigation and several reviews (6-10). Interestingly, the initial steps in the browning reaction and the nonenzymatic glycosylation reaction are essentially the same. However, it is not certain whether in vivo proteins undergo the final stages in the Maillard browning reaction.

Structural and functional diversity among proteins is enhanced by posttranslational modification, i.e., the covalent modification of amino acid residue(s) of the protein during or after the completion of the protein synthesis. Many of these reactions are precisely controlled by enzymes and cofactors. Nonenzymatic glycosylation, on the other hand, depends on the presence of high concentrations of reducing sugars, amino group accessibility, and protein half-life. Figure 1.1 provides a simple scheme for in vivo or in vitro nonenzymatic glycosylation of proteins. Reaction of ϵ-amino groups of lysines or the amino terminus of a protein with the acyclic form of glucose yields a Schiff-base intermediate. This aldimine, which is readily reversible, can undergo the practically irreversible Amadori rearrangement to a stable ketoamine derivative, which then cyclizes to the hemiketal structure. Unlike the browning reaction that requires nonphysiologic incubation conditions, nonenzymatic glycosylation of proteins takes place under physiologic conditions.

*The recently recommended (IUPAC-IUB) term is "glycation." The author, however, has chosen to use the most widely used term, "glycosylation."

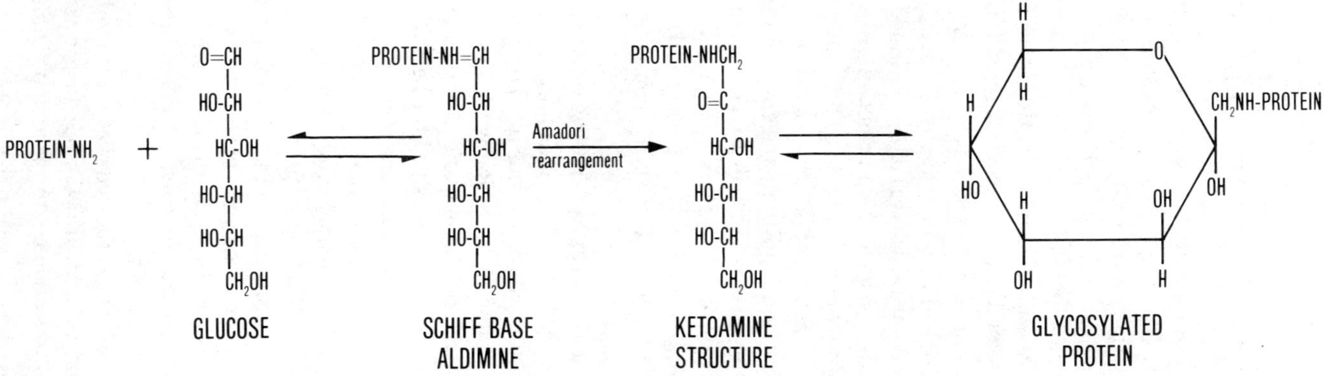

Figure 1.1 Scheme for nonenzymatic glycosylation reaction.

III. DISCOVERY OF GLYCOSYLATED HEMOGLOBINS

During the 1950s, several investigators focused their research on the electrophoretic and chromatographic heterogeneities of hemoglobins in human red cells; these studies have been reviewed before in great detail (11,12). Kunkel and Wallenius (13) reported in *Science* in 1955 the separation of minor fractions from human adult hemoglobin by starch block electrophoresis. Later studies in other laboratories utilizing Amberlite IRC-50 or carboxymethyl cellulose cation exchange chromatography have confirmed this apparent heterogeneity of the hemoglobins in human red cells (14-18). In 1959, Clegg and Schroeder (18), utilizing IRC-50 chromatography, demonstrated the presence of up to five minor components, which was later confirmed by Schnek and Schroeder (19). These authors named them hemoglobins A_{Ia}, A_{Ib}, A_{Ic}, A_{Id}, and A_{Ie} according to the order in which these hemoglobins were eluted from IRC-50 columns. The major hemoglobin components were termed Hb A_{II} and a less separated Hb A_{III} representing Hb A_o and Hb A_2, respectively, according to the present nomenclature system. The Hb A_{Ia+b} (Hb A_{Ia} and Hb A_{Ib} were not completely separated from each other) fraction was about 1.9%; Hb A_{Ic}, 6.1%; Hb A_{Id}, 1.6%; Hb A_{Ie}, 5.6%; Hb A_{II}, 78.0%; and Hb A_{III}, 7.0% in a normal adult. Thus, it became apparent that Hb A_{Ic} constituted the major portion of the total Hb A_I (Hb A_{Ia+b+c}).

Even before we learned that Hb A_{Ic} and few other minor hemoglobins are indeed glycosylated components, Huisman and Dozy (20) in 1962 first observed a two- to threefold increase in Hb A_I in four diabetic patients who were treated with tolbutamide. Later, in 1968, Rahbar (21) surveyed 1200 patients in Tehran University hospitals and found two diabetic patients who showed an abnormal pattern on agar gel electrophoresis of the hemoglobins. Subsequently, Rahbar and his co-workers (22) also examined another 47 diabetic patients and detected the same abnormal electrophoretic pattern in each case. In addition, they showed that the unusually increased component in the diabetics has the same electrophoretic and chromatographic properties as Hb A_{Ic}, and they observed a twofold increase (compared to normal controls) in chromatographically separated Hb A_{Ic} (21). Since then, similar observations were made in numerous laboratories. Such an increase in Hb A_{Ic} in diabetic patients could be easily explained by the information provided by concurrent and subsequent structural analyses done in various laboratories.

Holmquist and Schroeder (23) showed that the only difference between Hb A_{Ic} and Hb A_o was that an unidentified group (suggested a long-chain aromatic aldehyde or ketone) was attached to the amino-terminal valine of the β chains, presumably through a Schiff base linkage. Subsequently, Bookchin and

Gallop (24) have confirmed that a hexose was linked to the amino-terminal groups of both the β chains. It took another 10 years to identify completely most of the other minor Hbs (6,24). Adducts formed with glucose and phosphorylated glycolytic intermediates were identified. The β-chain amino terminus, the α-chain amino terminus, and the ε-amino groups of lysyl residues were shown to participate in the nonenzymatic glycosylation process (6,25, 26). Furthermore, similar glycosylated hemoglobins were shown to be present in newborn infants and in various hemoglobinopathies and formed from fetal hemoglobin (27) and various hemoglobin variants (28). The levels of the various glycosylated components, irrespective of the fact that they were formed from normal adult, fetal, or abnormal Hbs, were greatly influenced by diabetes and hemolytic anemia. Glycosylated hemoglobin levels were shown to directly reflect the time-averaged glucose levels for the preceding 2-3 months. Thus, these measurements have gained wide acceptance as an index of metabolic control of diabetes (29-32). Lately, numerous other proteins were shown to be glycosylated, the degree of glycosylation depending on intracellular glucose concentration and the half-life of the protein (33-39). The secondary sequelae of diabetes may be due to the protein modifications by glycosylation, which in many instances alter their structural and functional characteristics and even their turnover, and glycosylated hemoglobin may serve as a model for the development of the sequelae of diabetes.

REFERENCES

1. L. C. Maillard, *C. R. Acad. Sci., 154::* 66 (1912).
2. L. C. Maillard, *Ann. Chim., 6:* 258 (1918).
3. M. Saltmarch and T. P. Labuza, *Diabetes, 31* (Suppl. 3): 29 (1982).
4. V. Friedman, *Diabetes, 31* (Suppl. 3): 5 (1982).
5. P. A. Finot, *Diabetes, 31* (Suppl. 3): 22 (1982).
6. H. F. Bunn, K. H. Gabbay, and P. M. Gallop, *Science, 200:* 21 (1978).
7. A. Cerami and R. J. Koenig, *Trends Biochem. Sci., 3:* 73 (1978).
8. T. K. Mayer and Z. R. Freedman, *Clin. Chim. Acta, 127:* 147 (1983).
9. *Diabetes, 31* (Suppl. 3): (1982), proceedings of a conference on nonenzymatic glycosylation and browning reactions: their relevance to diabetes mellitus.
10. H. F. Bunn, *Am. J. Med., 70:* 325 (1981).
11. T. H. J. Huisman and J. H. P. Jonxis, *The Hemoglobinopathies: Techniques of Identification,* Marcel Dekker, New York (1977).
12. W. A. Schroeder and T. H. J. Huisman, *The Chromatography of Hemoglobin,* Marcel Dekker, New York (1980).

13. H. G. Kunkel and G. Wallenius, *Science, 122:* 288 (1955).
14. M. Morrison and J. L. Cook, *Fed. Proc., 16:* 765 (1957).
15. T. H. J. Huisman, E. A. Martis, and A. Dozy, *J. Lab. Clin. Med., 52:* 312 (1958).
16. D. W. Allen, W. A. Schroeder, and J. Balog, *J. Am. Chem. Soc., 80:* 1628 (1958).
17. F. J. Gutter, E. A. Peterson, and H. A. Sober, *Arch. Biochem. Biophys., 80:* 353 (1959).
18. M. D. Clegg and W. A. Schroeder, *J. Am. Chem. Soc., 81:* 6065 (1959).
19. A. G. Schnek and W. A. Schroeder, *J. Am. Chem. Soc., 83:* 1472 (1961).
20. T. H. J. Huisman and A. Dozy, *J. Lab. Clin. Med., 60:* 302 (1962).
21. S. Rahbar, *Clin. Chim. Acta, 22:* 296 (1968).
22. S. Rahbar, O. Blumenfeld, and H. M. Ranney, *Biochem. Biophys. Res. Comm., 36:* 838 (1969).
23. W. R. Holmquist and W. A. Schroeder, *Biochemistry, 5:* 2489 (1966).
24. R. M. Bookchin and P. M. Gallop, *Biochem, Biophys. Res. Commun., 32:* 86 (1968).
25. E. C. Abraham, M. Stallings, A. Abraham, and R. Clardy, *Biochim. Biophys. Acta, 744:* 335 (1983).
26. R. Shapiro, M. J. McManus, C. Zalut, and H. F. Bunn, *J. Biol Chem., 255:* 3120 (1980).
27. E. C. Abraham, *Biochim. Biophys. Acta, 667:* 168 (1981).
28. E. C. Abraham, M. Stallings, B. F. Cameron, and T. H. J. Huisman, *Biochim. Biophys. Acta, 625:* 109 (1980).
29. B. Gonen, A. H. Rubenstein, H. Rockman, S. P. Tanega, and D. L. Hortwitz, *Lancet, 2:* 734 (1977).
30. E. C. Abraham, T. A. Huff, N. D. Cope, J. B. Wilson, Jr., E. D. Bransome, Jr., and T. H. J. Huisman, *Diabetes, 27:* 931 (1978).
31. D. E. Goldstein, K. M. Parker, J. D. England, J. E. England, Jr., H. M. Wiedmeyer, S. S. Rawlings, R. Hess, R. R. Little, J. F. Simonds, and R P. Breyfogle, *Diabetes, 31* (Suppl. 3): 70 (1982).
32. L. Jovanovic and C. E. Peterson, *Am. J. Med., 70:* 331 (1981).
33. V. J. Stevens, C. A. Rouzer, V. M. Monnier, and A. Cerami, *Proc. Natl. Acad. Sci., USA, 75:* 2918 (1978).
34. J. L. Witztum, M. Fisher, T. Pietro, U. P. Steinbrecher, and R. L. Elam, *Diabetes, 31:* 1029 (1982).
35. J. L. Witztum, M. Mahoney, M. J. Branks, M. Fisher, R. L. Elam, and D. Steinberg, *Diabetes, 31:* 283 (1982).
36. H. F. Bunn, S. H. Chiou, L. T. Chylack, and W. H. Tung, *J. Biol. Chem., 256:* 5176 (1981).
37. J. A. Miller, E. Gravallese, and H. F. Bunn, *J. Clin. Invest., 65:* 896 (1980).
38. J. F. Day, S. R. Thorpe, and J. W. Baynes, *J. Biol. Chem., 254:* 595 (1979).
39. D. E. McMillan and S. M. Brooks, *Diabetes, 31* (Suppl. 3): 64 (1982).

2

The Structure and Function of Hemoglobin

I. THE HEME GROUP

A. Structure and Biosynthesis

The prosthetic group of hemoglobin, heme, is a ferroprotoporphyrin IX in which the iron atom is located at the center of the porphyrin ring (Fig. 2.1). The heme disc measures 14 × 17 Å. The porphyrin ring itself is formed from four pyrroles that are linked by methene bridges. Succinic acid and glycine are the precursors of pyrrole rings (1,2). The activated forms of these two compounds combine to form δ-aminolevulinic acid (ALA) in the presence of ALA synthetase and pyridoxal phosphate. This reaction is the rate-limiting step in heme synthesis. δ-Aminolevulinic dehydrase catalyzes the condensation of two molecules of ALA to porphobilinogen, which is basically a pyrrole ring structure. The biosynthetic pathway for the heme from porphobilinogen proceeds through a series of steps. The four porphyrin rings in heme have altogether four methyl, two vinyl, and two propionic acid groups. These groups can be arranged in a number of ways; this results in the existence of several forms of protoporphyrins. The heme present in hemoglobin has been termed protoporphyrin IX (Fig. 2.1).

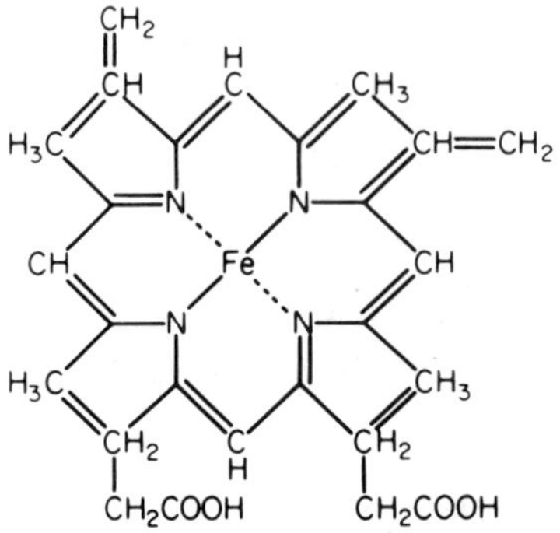

Figure 2.1 The structure of ferroprotoporphyrin IX (heme) in hemoglobin.

B. The Heme as an Oxygen Carrier

The iron in hemoglobin, but neither the inorganic iron nor the free heme, is capable of reversible combination with molecular oxygen. This is possible only if the heme is maintained in the ferrous form in an uncharged hydrophobic surrounding. In fact, on the surface of each polypeptide there is a pocket into which the heme is deeply buried (Figs. 2.2 and 2.3). The polypeptide chain that surrounds the heme is rich in aromatic side chains and other residues, providing a hydrophobic environment for the heme (1,3-6). Each prosthetic group, namely, heme, consists of a protoporphyrin IX ring with a Fe^{2+} atom held in the center of the ring by coordination with the four nitrogen atoms of the porphyrin structure. The fifth and the sixth coordination positions of the iron atom are available for ligand binding, one on each side of the porphyrin ring. The fifth coordination position of the iron atom is linked to the polypeptide chain through linkage of the iron with the imidazole nitrogen of the so-called proximal histidine (7-9), which is residue number 87 in the α chain and 92 in both β and γ chains. The sixth coordination position is occupied by a ligand in the ligand form and unoccupied in the nonligand form. It seems possible that the region of the E helix directly opposite the sixth coordination position of the iron atom, particularly the histidine residue (distal histidine) at this site, is also important in the reversible combination of oxygen with the iron.

The heme itself is not a disc but resembles a flattened pyramid, the opening formed by the four nitrogen atoms of the pyrrole rings pointing toward the proximal histidine. The Fe^{2+} atom in the reduced state is too large

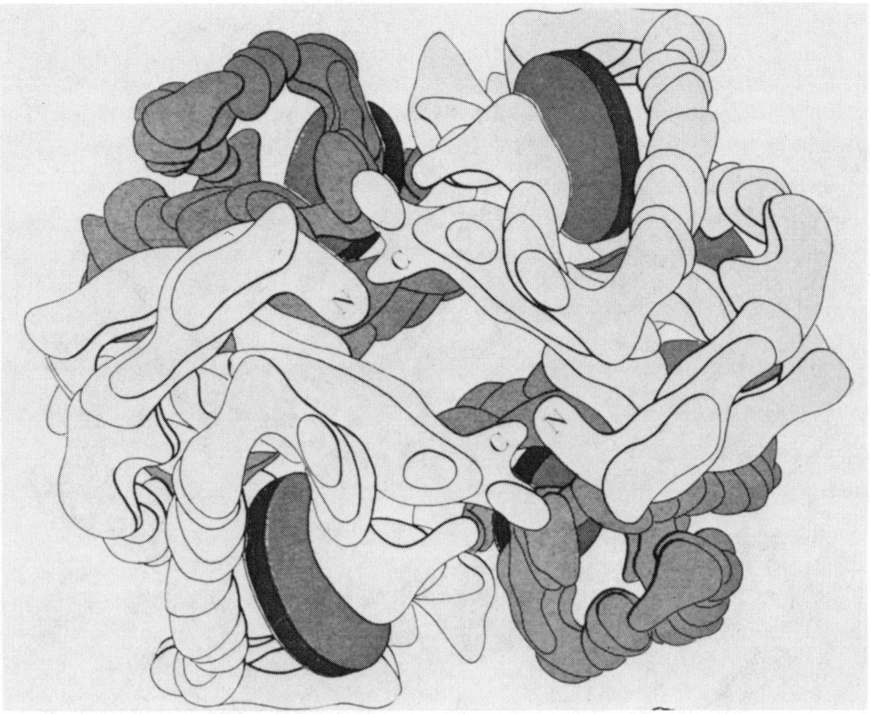

Figure 2.2 The model of hemoglobin at low resolution. The α chains in this model are white and the β chains are black. The binding site for 23-diphosphoglycerate (2,3-DPG) is in the central cavity of the molecule. From Perutz (9) by permission of the W. H. Freeman and Company Publishers for *Scientific American.*

to fit into the central cavity of the porphyrin ring, and so it lies at the very top of this flat pyramid. Once the oxygen molecule becomes attached, the ferrous iron shares an electron with it and reduces its volume by 13%. The oxygen-linked iron atom can now slip into the plane of the porphyrin, at the same time pulling the proximal histidine with it (10). The conformational changes that take place while going from reduced state to oxy state are, in fact, initiated by this movement of the proximal histidine. Apart from the iron-protein bond, other linkages between the heme and the protein exist that confer stability on the heme-protein complex. The propionic acid side chains of the porphyrin

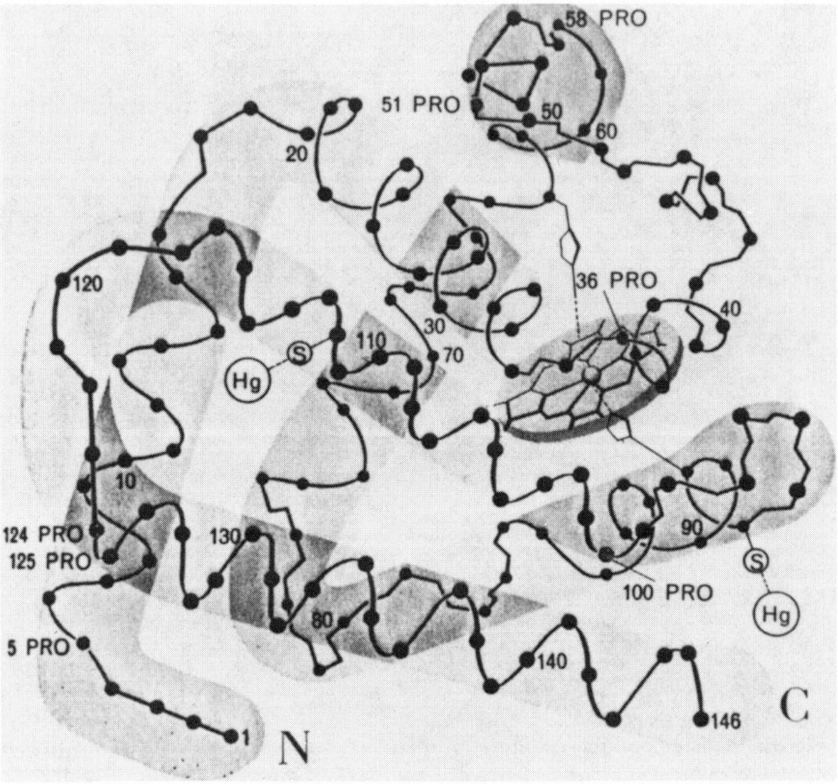

Figure 2.3 The β chain of human hemoglobin. Every tenth amino acid and every proline are marked. The point of attachment of heme is also clearly shown. From Perutz (9) by permission of the W. H. Freeman and Company Publishers for *Scientific American.*

ring are on the exterior of the Hb molecule, and one of them is probably linked to an arginine residue on the polypeptide chains. Hydrophobic interaction exists between the vinyl side chains of the porphyrin ring and the hydrophobic side chains of the aromatic amino acids that surround them.

In addition to oxygen, other compounds, such as nitric oxide and carbon monoxide, are also able to combine with the ferrous atom of hemoglobin (6). Carbon monoxide is attached more firmly than oxygen. Once carboxyhemoglobin is formed, the oxygen does not displace carbon monoxide to any extent, and this is the molecular basis of carbon monoxide poisoning. The heme, under certain conditions, can form reversible or irreversible hemochromogens. Hemochromogens are combinations of heme and any nitrogenous compound such as pyridine (11). The formation of reversible hemochromogens is the initial step in the subsequent formation of irreversible hemochromogens and the precipitation in the form of Heinz bodies. If hemoglobin becomes oxidized to the ferric state, methemoglobin is formed. Methemoglobin cannot take up oxygen, but it can form linkages with radicals such as cyanide and fluoride.

II. THE PROTEIN STRUCTURE

A. The Primary Structure: General Considerations

The primary structure, i.e., the amino acid sequence of the polypeptide chains (α, β, γ, δ, etc), is due to linking of the amino acid residues by covalent peptide bonds.

Amino Acids

Amino acids are the basic structural units of proteins. An amino acid consists of an amino group, a carboxyl group, a hydrogen atom, and a distinctive R group (side chain) bond to a carbon atom, which is called the α-carbon (Fig. 2.4). Amino acids in solution at neutral pH are predominantly dipolar ions. In the dipolar form, the amino group is protonated ($-NH_3^+$), and the carboxyl group is dissociated ($-COO^-$). The ionization state of an amino acid varies with pH and the pK values of the α-COOH, α-NH_2, and the R groups. The tetrahedral array of four different groups about the α-carbon confers optical activity on the amino acids; both L isomers and D isomers are present. Only the L-amino acids are the constituents of proteins.

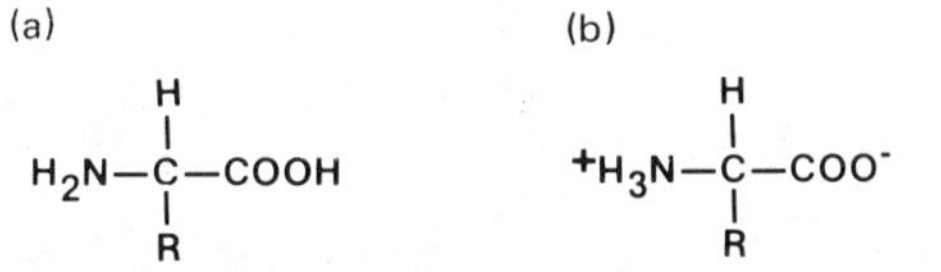

Figure 2.4 The structure of the un-ionized (a) and the zwitterion (b) forms of an amino acid.

Table 2.1 Classification and Abbreviations for Amino Acids

Amino acid	Side chain characteristic	Three-letter abbreviations	One-letter symbol
Alanine	Hydrophobic (aliphatic)	Ala	A
Valine	Hydrophobic (aliphatic)	Val	V
Glycine	Hydrophobic (aliphatic)	Gly	G
Leucine	Hydrophobic (sliphatic)	Leu	L
Isoleucine	Hydrophobic (aliphatic)	Ile	I
Phenylalanine	Hydrophobic (aromatic)	Phe	F
Tyrosine	Hydrophobic (aromatic)	Tyr	Y
Tryptophan	Hydrophobic (aromatic)	Trp	W
Methionine	Hydrophobic (sulfur-containing)	Met	M
Cysteine	Hydrophobic (sulfur-containing)	Cys	C
Proline	Hydrophobic (imino acid)	Pro	P
Serine	Uncharged polar (aliphatic hydroxyl)	Ser	S
Threonine	Uncharged polar (aliphatic hydroxyl)	Thr	T
Asparagine	Uncharged polar (amide)	Asn	N
Glutamine	Uncharged polar (amide)	Glu	Q
Aspartic acid	Hydrophilic (acidic)	Asp	D
Glutamic acid	Hydrophilic (acidic)	Glu	E

Table 2.1 (continued)

Amino acid	Side chain characteristic	Three-letter abbreviations	One-letter symbol
Arginine	Hydrophilic (basic)	Arg	R
Lysine	Hydrophilic (basic)	Lys	K
Histidine	Hydrophilic (basic)	His	H

Twenty different kinds of side chains, and thus 20 different amino acids, are commonly found in proteins. Classification of amino acids is done on the basis of the side chain characteristics. They are generally classified as amino acids with hydrophilic side chains, uncharged polar side chains, and hydrophobic side chains (Table 2.1). The classification may be done in a more detailed manner as amino acids having aliphatic, aliphatic hydroxyl, aromatic, basic, acidic, amide, or sulfur-containing side chains (Table 2.1).

The hydrophilic amino acid residues make the molecule water-soluble. Such amino acid residues are generally found on the surface or lining of the central cavity of the hemoglobin molecule. An aqueous solution surrounding the protein molecule would not be repelled at the site of a hydrophilic amino acid side chain, and, as a result, the protein is made soluble. The hydrophobic amino acid residues are found mostly in the interior of the molecule and also lining the heme pocket.

The Peptide Link

The peptide link or bond (Fig. 2.5) is formed by joining the α-carboxyl group of one amino acid to the α-amino group of another amino acid with the elimination of a water molecule. The equilibrium of this reaction forming a dipeptide lies far on the side of hydrolysis rather than synthesis. Therefore, the synthesis of a peptide, chemically or biologically, requires input of energy.

The first amino acid in a polypeptide chain is called the amino-terminal or N-terminal residue. Likewise, the last residue is called carboxy-terminal or C-terminal residue. By convention, the N-terminal residue of the sequence is placed at the left. Once an amino acid has been incorporated into a peptide chain, it is then referred to as an amino acid residue. It is convenient to name

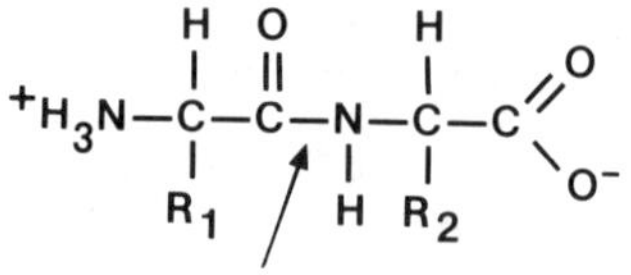

Figure 2.5 A peptide bond.

these by a shorthand, e.g., glutamyl for a glutamic acid residue or lysyl for a lysine residue, or simply Glu or Lys, respectively (Table 2.1). For convenience, each amino acid has been assigned a single letter as well (Table 2.1).

The polypeptide backbone is merely repetitive. The only allowable variability occurs when the pyrrolidine ring of proline is incorporated into the polypeptide chain. The chemical and the physical properties of the polypeptide chain are controlled by their side chain characteristics. The net charge on the polypeptide chain is greatly influenced by the intrinsic pK values of the various basic and acidic groups (Table 2.2). It should be pointed out that ionization of such groups in a polypeptide chain may show variations from protein to protein.

Table 2.2 pK Values for Acidic and Basic Groups on Proteins

Groups	pK values (range)
α-Carboxyl	3.0- 3.2
β-Carboxyl	3.0- 4.7
γ-Carboxyl	~4.4
Imidazolium	5.6- 7.0
α-Amino	7.6- 8.4
ε-Amino	9.4-10.6
Guanidinium	11.6-12.6
Phenolic hydroxyl	9.8-10.4
Sulfhydryl	~8-9

Amino Acid Sequence

Amino acids in a protein are arranged in a definite order that appears to be important to the functions of the molecule. In fact, the primary structure dictates the secondary and tertiary structures and thus the function. In 1953, Frederick Sanger determined the amino acid sequence of insulin. This work is a landmark in biochemistry because it showed for the first time that a protein has a definite amino acid sequence. Indeed, the complete amino acid sequences of several hundreds of proteins, including numerous hemoglobins, are known. It is a well-established fact that amino acid sequences are genetically determined. The sequence of nucleotides in DNA specifies a complementary sequence of nucleotides in RNA, which specifies the amino acid sequence of a polypeptide chain.

The methods of sequencing, including several microsequencing approaches, have been reviewed in great detail in other reports (4,12-14) and some general concepts are summarized here.

Prerequisite considerations are the following:

1. Purity of the protein
2. Amount of the protein required
3. Analytical considerations
   a. Physical methods
   b. Chemical methods
      i. N-terminal and C-terminal analyses
      ii. Amino acid composition

Preparative treatments are the following:

1. Removal of prosthetic groups
2. Cleavage of disulfide bonds and blockage of sulfhydryl groups and other groups, if necessary
3. Separation of subunits
4. Chemical and/or enzymatic cleavage of the polypeptide chain
5. Separation of the peptides

Methods of sequence analysis are the following:

1. The substrative method of Konigsberg
2. The Edman method
3. The dansyl-Edman method

4. The method of DABITC/PITC–double coupling
5. Mass spectral methods

The assignment of the position of the disulfide bridges and of the point of the linkage of prosthetic groups and carbohydrate moieties are even more challenging and require special attention in the sequencing process. The presence of a blocking group at the N-terminal residue makes it difficult to determine the number of polypeptide chains and is an effective obstacle to the application of a degradative method such as the Edman procedure. A variety of causes, such as acetylation, glycosylation (nonenzymatic), formylation, and cyclization, may contribute to the blocking of the N-terminal amino acid.

B. The Primary Structures of the α, β, γ, and δ Chains

Several structurally different hemoglobin chains are synthesized from the time of conception to adult life. The polypeptide chains of human hemoglobins have been named according to the Greek alphabets: alpha (α), beta (β), gamma (γ), delta (δ), epsilon (ϵ), and zeta (ζ). The polypeptide chain compositions of the major adult hemoglobin (Hb A); fetal hemoglobin (Hb F); Hb A_2; and the embryonic hemoglobins Grower 1, Grower 2, and Portland I are $\alpha_2\beta_2$, $\alpha_2\gamma_2$, $\alpha_2\delta_2$, $\alpha_2\epsilon_2$, $\gamma_2\epsilon_2$, and $\zeta_2\gamma_2$, respectively (1,4,5).

The amino acid sequence of the α and β chains of Hb A were determined in the early 1960s. The α chain contains 141 amino acid residues, whereas β, γ, and δ chains have 146. The primary structure of the γ chain of Hb F from newborn was determined in 1963. The γ chain and the β chain differ in 39 positions. The presence of the four isoleucyl residues is a distinct characteristic of Hb F. The tryptophanyl residue in position 130 (tyrosine in the β chain) is responsible for the well-known "tryptophan notch" at 289.8 nm of the ultraviolet spectrum of Hb F. There are two types of γ chains that differ in one position, namely, position 136, which is occupied by a glycyl residue in the $^G\gamma$ chain and by an alanyl residue in the $^A\gamma$ chain. The primary structures of the β chain and the δ chain differ in 10 positions.

Hemoglobin A comprises about 97% of the hemoglobin of the adult, Hb A_2 2.5%, and Hb F the remaining. Small amounts of β chains are present in the fetus during the second trimester of pregnancy. After birth, β and δ chains replace γ chains. The level of Hb F at birth varies between 60 and 90% and is usually less than 2% in 6-month-old infants. Embryonic hemoglobins have been observed in young embryos not older than 12 weeks.

C. The Secondary and Tertiary Structures

In hemoglobin and myoglobin, about 80% of each polypeptide chain is in the α-helical structure, which was predicted by Pauling and Corey and subsequently seen in x-ray crystallography. The α-helix has 3.6 amino acid residues per turn of the helix with a 1.5 Å translational movement along the helical axis per residue. The helix is stabilized by hydrogen bonding between amino acids lying above or below each other in adjacent turns, a carbonyl (CO) group of one amino acid being bonded to an imino (NH) group four residues further down. Such hydrogen bonds are relatively weak and are readily disrupted by heat and denaturing agents.

The helix is a firm, straight structure. However, in order to achieve the globular shape of the hemoglobin molecule, it is necessary for the helix to bend and fold in a complex but fixed pattern. The tertiary structure concerns the folding of the polypeptide chain and the helical structures. The β chain contains eight helical segments, termed A, B, C, D, E, F, G, and H; and the α chain has seven (D helix is absent). The helical segments are often joined by nonhelical segments, designated by the letters of the adjoining helices (EF, FG, GH, etc). Nonhelical segments are also found at the amino-terminal end (NA) and carboxy-terminal end (HC). The tertiary structure is stabilized by hydrophobic bonds in the interior of the polypeptide, by similar interactions around the heme, and by weak interactions of the van der Waals type. Polar residues, such as the basic groups of histidine, lysine, and arginine and the acidic groups of aspartic and glutamic acid, are situated on the outer surface of the folded polypeptide and interact freely with the solvent. The presence of proline residues can disrupt the helical structure by presumably forming a cyclic structure between the side chain of this amino acid and its own amide nitrogen. For this reason, prolyl residues mainly occur in the amino-terminal region of an α helix. The heme group in both α and β chains is buried in a pocket of hydrophobic residues of the B, C, E, F, G, and H helices, and of the CD and FG interhelical segments.

D. The Quaternary Structure

The quaternary structure in hemoglobin arises from the organization of four different chains. The tetrameric structure is highly essential for normal function, i.e., the sigmoid oxygen dissociation curve, heme-heme interaction, and the Bohr effect. The forces holding the chains together are noncovalent in nature, and they are predominantly the van der Waals type with minimal involvement of hydrogen bonds and ionic interactions.

Detailed insight into the quaternary structure of hemoglobin was the result of the many observations from Perutz's laboratory (15-17). The contact between unlike chains are of two different types: the α_1-β_1 contact and the α_1-β_2 contact. Thirty-four residues, involving about 110 atoms, participate in the α_1-β_1 contact in contrast to only 19 residues and 80 atoms for the α_1-β_2 contact. Dissociation of the hemoglobin tetramer into dimers ($\alpha_2\beta_2 \rightleftharpoons 2\alpha\beta$) depends on factors such as the ligand at the iron atom, the Hb concentration, the electrolyte concentration, the pH, and the temperature. This symmetrical dissociation into dimers occurs at the α_1-β_2 contact. The α and β chain monomers are formed when dissociation occurs at α_1-β_1 contact below pH 4.9 or above pH 11.0.

Contacts between like chains ($\alpha_1\alpha_2$ or $\beta_1\beta_2$) are minimal by comparison with the contacts between unlike chains and are ionic in nature. An internal cavity (Fig. 2.2) lined by polar amino acids and filled with water separates the like chains from each other. When the hemoglobin is in the oxygenated form, no contacts are present between α chains. However, upon oxygenation, intra- and interchain salt bridges are formed. The presence of at least four pairs of salt bridges has been recognized in the deoxygenated tetramer. Moreover, one molecule of 2,3-diphosphoglycerate (2,3-DPG) fits between the two β chains in the deoxy configuration, and thus, provides additional contacts for stabilizing the quaternary structure of this configuration. The binding sites of 2,3-DPG on the β chain are Val NA_1 (1), His NA_2 (2), Lys EF_6 (82), and His H_{21} (143). It should be pointed out that blocking the Val NA_1 residue (acetylation, nonenzymatic glycosylation, etc.) disrupts the 2,3-DPG binding, leading to destabilization of the deoxy conformation. Of the 39 differences between β and γ chains, two are part of the heme contact and four are part of the α_1-β_1 contact. The replacement in the α_1-β_1 contact of Hb F are responsible for the relatively slow dissociation of $\alpha\gamma$ dimer to α and γ monomers. Moreover, the substitution of His H_{21} (residue 143) in the β chains with a Tyr residue in the γ chains prevents the binding of 2,3-DPG to Hb F with an apparent increase in oxygen affinity of fetal blood.

III. FUNCTIONAL ASPECTS OF HEMOGLOBIN: OXYGENATION

A. General Characteristics

Oxygenation is the reversible combination of oxygen with hemoglobin. Most of the very early workers in this field visualized the reaction of hemoglobin with oxygen as a simple process represented by the reaction

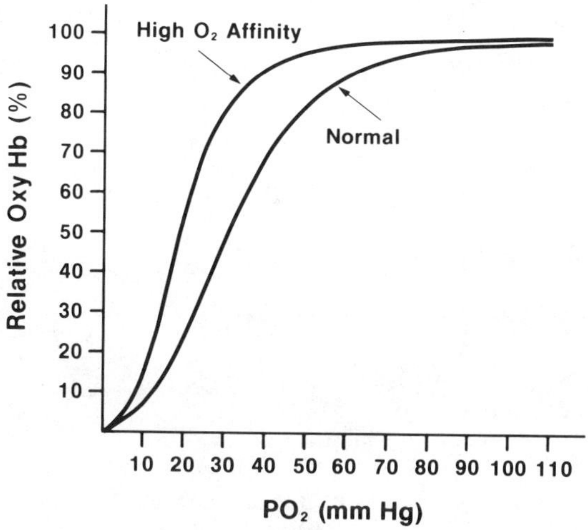

Figure 2.6 Oxyhemoglobin dissociation curves of a normal blood sample and a blood sample with high oxygen affinity. The curves were obtained at 37°C with a HEM-O-SCAN (American Instrument Company, Silver Spring, MD).

$$Hb + O_2 \rightleftharpoons HbO_2$$

Contrary to this, in 1904 Bohr and co-workers (18) and later others showed that when the fraction of oxygenated hemoglobin was plotted against the partial pressure of oxygen, the curve (Fig. 2.6, and also see Fig. 3.14) had a sigmoid shape as compared to hyperbolic shape that would have resulted from the above reaction. The theoretical treatments developed by Hill in 1910 (19) and Adair in 1925 (20) were leading steps for a better understanding of the oxygenation reaction. According to Hill, if the reaction between oxygen and hemoglobin were represented as

$$Hb + n\,O_2 \rightleftharpoons Hb(O_2)_n$$

the equilibrium constant of the above reaction would be

$$K = \frac{[Hb(O_2)_n]}{[Hb]\ [O_2]_n}$$

Simple rearrangement of the above equation leads to the following expression where Y is the fractional saturation:

$$Y = \frac{[Hb(O_2)_n]}{[Hb] + [Hb(O_2)_n]} = \frac{K(pO_2)^n}{1 + K(pO_2)^n}$$

The logarithmic form of the above equation is

$$\log\left(\frac{Y}{1 - Y}\right) = n \log(pO_2) + \log K$$

Today we see that Hill's empirical equation has no physical significance, but it is quite useful, as it fits the experimental data well for hemoglobins at values of Y between 0.1 and 0.9. The parameters K, P_{50} (the partial pressure of oxygen at 50% saturation), and n (the Hill coefficient) serve to characterize the equilibrium and to compare different hemoglobins under various conditions. The exponent n is closely related to the extent of the cooperative interactions (the interaction energy) in the system. For mammalian hemoglobins, the value of n, when the value of pO_2 is close to P_{50}, is about 3. The P_{50} or $\log(P_{50})$ is widely used as a measure of oxygen affinity. At 50% saturation [when $\log(P_{50})$ equals $-(\log K/n)$], $\log(P_{50})$ can be used as a measure of K.

Adair, in 1925 (20) found that there were four hemes in each hemoglobin molecule and proposed four sequential addition reactions for a more reasonable understanding of the oxygenation reaction. The Adair model describes the reactions of hemoglobin in terms of individual equilibrium and kinetic constants corresponding to the four hemes. The scheme is as follows

$$Hb_4 + O_2 \underset{k_1}{\overset{k_1'}{\rightleftharpoons}} Hb_4O_2 \qquad K_1 = k_1'/k_1$$

$$Hb_4O_2 + O_2 \underset{k_2}{\overset{k_2'}{\rightleftharpoons}} Hb_4(O_2)_2 \qquad K_2 = k_2'/k_2$$

$$Hb_4(O_2)_2 + O_2 \underset{k_3}{\overset{k_3'}{\rightleftharpoons}} Hb_4(O_2)_3 \qquad K_3 = k_3'/k_3$$

$$Hb_4(O_2)_3 + O_2 \underset{k_4}{\overset{k_4'}{\rightleftharpoons}} Hb_4(O_2)_4 \qquad K_4 = k_4'/k_4$$

where K, k′, and k are the equilibrium constant, the combination velocity constant, and the dissociation velocity constant, respectively. The Adair model still finds application as a formal model in hemoglobin reactions even though all the aspects of equilibria and kinetics of hemoglobin cannot be accommodated in its framework. The difficult problem of determining these individual constants was attacked by Gibson and his collaborators (21,22).

B. The Bohr Effect

The variation of oxygen affinity with pH was discovered by Bohr et al. (18) in 1904 when they demonstrated that the changes in the partial pressure of carbon dioxide influence the oxygen equilibrium of blood. Ten years later, Christiansen et al. (23) reported the reciprocal effect, that oxygenated blood absorbed less carbon dioxide than deoxygenated blood. These two effects are now commonly called the "Bohr effect." As first pointed out by Henderson (24), the Bohr effect is the expression of a functional interaction between oxygen binding sites and ionizable groups. In practical terms, the change in oxygen affinity, measured by P_{50} or $\log(P_{50})$, with change in pH is known as the oxygenation Bohr effect. This change observed in the region of pH 6 to 9 is termed the normal or the "alkaline" Bohr effect, and the change noted in the pH region below 6 is called the reverse or the "acid" Bohr effect. Physiologically, the Bohr effect means that the presence of higher levels of acidic metabolites and CO_2 in the capillaries of metabolically active tissue promotes the release of oxygen from oxyhemoglobin.

The relation between the change in oxygen affinity with pH and the number of Bohr protons released or bound upon oxygenation of hemoglobin was put forward by Wyman (25) as

$$\frac{\Delta \log(P_{50})}{\Delta \mathrm{pH}} = \Delta x$$

where Δx is the difference in the number of protons bound by oxy- and deoxy-Hb per mole of heme at any given pH. The alkaline Bohr effect is synchronous with the oxygenation reaction, and the liberation of Bohr protons is exactly proportional to the amount of oxygen taken up. Rossi-Bernardi and Roughton (26) measured the number of protons released or bound during oxygenation, and the results indicated the presence of at least three alkaline Bohr groups per Hb tetramer. Subsequent studies in a number of laboratories, including the landmark report by Perutz (10), have indicated that about 50% of the alkaline Bohr effect appears to be due to the salt bridge between the imidazole side chain of histidine 146 (HC3) of the β chain and the γ-carboxyl side chain of aspartic acid 94 (FG1) of the β chain. The salt bridges between the NH_2 groups of the amino-terminal valyl residues and the COOH- groups of the carboxy-terminal arginyl residues are responsible for the remainder of the effect.

Carbon dioxide, another regulator of oxygen transport, binds to the amino groups at the NH_2-terminal ends of the four polypeptide chains through carbamate formation. The presence of increased concentration of CO_2 will tend to fix the tetramer in the deoxy conformation by preferentially reacting with deoxy-Hb. Thus, the reduced Hb when linked with CO_2 will be less avid for oxygen and will tend to release more oxygen. Since N-terminal valine serves as a binding site for both CO_2 and H^+, these two must compete for the same site. In addition, CO_2 must compete with the organic phosphate, 2,3-DPG for the above site.

C. 2,3-Diphosphoglycerate and Oxygenation

A glycolytic intermediate, namely, 2,3-DPG (the structure of this compound shown in Fig. 2.7), exists with hemoglobin in the red cell in equimolar concentrations. Chanutin and Churnish (27) and Benesch and collaborators (28-30) have observed that the oxygen affinity of hemoglobin is strongly influenced

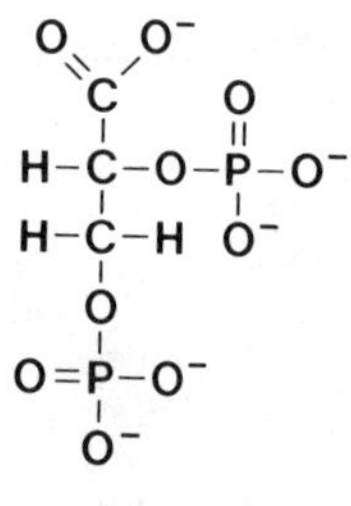

Figure 2.7 The structure of 2,3-diphosphoglycerate (2,3-DPG).

by this organic phosphate. There is a decrease in the oxygen affinity as 2,3-DPG increases (see Fig. 3.6 and Table 3.3). In fact, in the absence of 2,3-DPG, the P_{50} of hemoglobin is 1 torr, which is increased to 26 torr in the presence of normal level of 2,3-DPG. 2,3-Diphosphoglycerate is preferentially but reversibly bound to deoxyhemoglobin. The binding of oxygen and 2,3-DPG to hemoglobin is mutually exclusive. The negatively charged groups on this compound form salt bonds with positively charged residues on the two β chains at the entrance to the central cavity of the hemoglobin molecule. The extra bridges provided by 2,3-DPG stabilizes the quaternary structure more toward the deoxy (tense) conformation. Upon oxygenation, the distance between the α-amino groups of Val NA_1 of the β chains increases from 16 to 20 Å, and no contact can be made with 2,3-DPG (10). At this point, the H helices in the two β chains begin closing, and the 2,3-DPG molecule is expelled from the central cavity. As mentioned earlier, due to the replacement of residue 143 (BH21), which is near the central cavity, with a seryl residue in the γ chain, the oxygen affinity of cord blood erythrocytes is considerably higher than that of adult red blood cells.

IV. THE HEMOGLOBINOPATHIES

According to Weatherall and Clegg (5), the hemoglobinopathies may be classified as (a) hemoglobin variants having altered structure of globin chains occurring with or without any physiological or clinical abnormality, (b) inherited defects in the rate of synthesis of one or more of the globin chains or the thalassemias, (c) disorders with an inherited abnormality of both the structure and the rate of synthesis of the globin chains, generally giving the clinical picture of thalassemia, and (d) a genetic failure of the normal neonatal switch from fetal to adult hemoglobin known as hereditary persistence of fetal hemoglobin (HPFH), that usually shows no hematological or clinical abnormality. Several books and monographs have appeared during the last decade providing detailed discussion of the various hemoglobinopathies (1,3-5). It is beyond the scope of this book to discuss every aspect of this vast area.

A. Hemoglobin Variants

More than 300 structural variants of hemoglobin have been detected. The majority of the variants result from single amino acid (single base on the genetic code) substitutions. Other molecular mechanisms may result in rare variants with shortened polypeptide chains, elongated chains, and fusion chains.

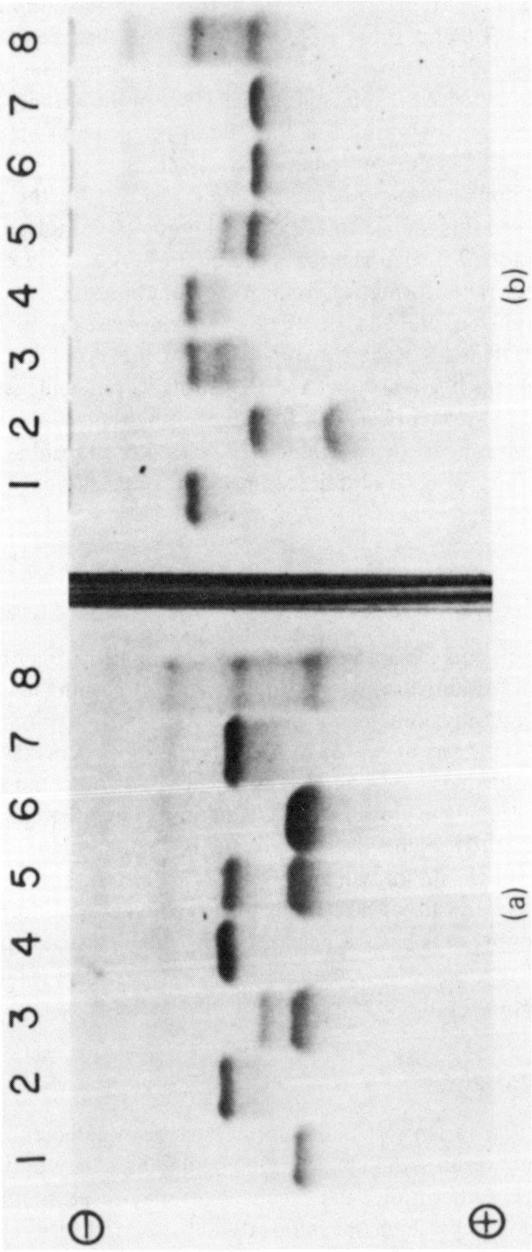

Figure 2.8 Cellulose-acetate electrophoresis of hemoglobins: (a) 1, A-β-thalassemia; 2, SS; 3, A-HPFH; 4, SS; 5, AS; 6, AA; 7, SS; 8, standard A-F-S-C. (b) 1, SS; 2, AN-Baltimore; 3, S-β^+-thalassemia; 4, S-HPFH; 5, A-HPFH; 6, A-β-thalassemia; 7, AA; 8, standard A-F-S-C. From Huisman and Jonxis (4).

Table 2.3 Some Common Hemoglobin Structural Variants

Hemoglobin variant	Substitution	Chain and position
S	Glu→Val	β6 (A3)
C	Glu→Lys	β6 (A3)
D-Punjab (Los Angeles)	Glu→Gln	β121 (GH4)
E	Glu→Lys	β26 (B8)
O-Arab	Glu→Lys	β126 (GH4)
N-Baltimore	Lys→Glu	β95 (FG2)
J-Baltimore	Gly→Asp	β16 (A13)

In most cases, the variants have been identified by electrophoretic techniques. Figure 2.8 shows cellulose acetate electrophoretic separation of some common variants. Structural variants may be grouped as methemoglobins, hemoglobins with increased or lowered oxygen affinity, and hemoglobins that tend to be unstable or may crystallize. Some commonly occurring variants, such as Hb S and Hb C (Table 2.3), and unstable hemoglobins may lead to hemolytic anemia; high affinity variants and hemoglobin M can cause cyanosis. A most popular and definitely simpler classification is based on differences in structure, i.e., the amino acid sequence of the various chains. A letter alphabet (Hb S, Hb C, Hb O, etc.) was originally used to describe each variant until these letters have been used up. It is now customary to designate a new hemoglobin by its place of discovery. The α, β, γ, and δ chain variants have been described. Table 2.3 summarizes the common structural variants; these are mainly β-chain variants.

B. The Sickling Disorders

Although the terms "sickle cell disease" and "sickling disorders" are used rather loosely, they are meant to include sickle cell anemia, which is the homozygous state for the sickle cell gene, and the heterozygous state for this gene in combination with either other structural hemoglobin variants or various types of thalassemia. The conditions that are included under sickling disorders are sickle cell anemia, Hb SD disease, Hb SC disease, Hb S-O Arab disease, Hb S-β-thalassemia, Hb S-α-thalassemia, and Hb S-HPFH. Sickle cell anemia has earned its reputation as the most severe of all, since homozygosity for Hb S (*SS*) is clinically severe with frequent episodes of pain crisis and red cell hemolysis resulting in chronic anemia. About 10% of Black Americans are heterozygous for this gene, which translates to about 1 in 600 having sickle cell anemia. The incidence is significantly higher in various parts of Africa. The disease is also found in Mediterranean countries as well as in Saudi Arabia and India. Sickle cell anemia is an inherited anomaly transmitted as a recessive gene.

Hemoglobin S differs from Hb A by the substitution of valine for glutamic acid at the sixth position of the β chain. Each known hemoglobin mutant characterized by a single amino acid change can be accounted for by a simple point mutation in the DNA encoding the β-globin sequence. In Hb S, a single point mutation in the DNA codon for glutamic acid appears to result in a base triplet that is transcribed into a mRNA that codes for valine. When the red cell containing this hemoglobin releases its oxygen, the cell loses its normal discoid shape to form a sickle shape. Upon reoxygenation, the red cell is reversed to its normal shape. The change from discoid to sickle shape is the consequence of intracellular hemoglobin gelation and crystallization or tactoid formation. It should be emphasized that complete deoxygenation need not be achieved for sickling to occur. When deoxygenation reaches a critical level, Hb S-containing cells will sickle. During sickling, a loss of intracellular water content and an increase in mean cell hemoglobin concentration (MCHC) take place. Even fully oxygenated blood from patients with sickle cell anemia may have some sickle-shaped cells. These are irreversibly sickled (deformed) cells (ISCs) presumably formed due to acquired membrane damage during repeated sickling-unsickling cycles. These cells generally contain relatively low levels of Hb F and do not seem to represent the scenescent cell population. The number of ISCs may vary from patient to patient, and an increase in these cells may lead to enhanced hemolysis (hemolytic anemia) and obstruction of microvasculature leading to organ damage. The sickling process increases the viscosity of the blood, which diminishes the blood flow rate and thus the oxygenation of the tissues.

Patients with sickle cell anemia and other sickling disorders are prone to intermittent episodes of sickle cell crises, i.e., vaso-occlusive hemolytic, aplastic, and sequestration episodes. An infant with sickle cell anemia is normally free of any clinical symptoms for the first 6 months. The simultaneous presence of another hemoglobin in the erythrocyte influences the gelation and thus the sickling. Hemoglobin D-Punjab and Hb O-Arab, for instances, promote it, and Hb F diminishes it. The influence of fetal hemoglobin may be particularly evident in Hb S-HPFH cases where Hb F levels of up to 30% are seen and it is evenly distributed over the red cells. In sickle cell anemia (*SS*) patients an average of only 8% (rarely more than 20%) Hb F is seen, and it is heterogenously distributed among the red cells. In any case, it is generally believed that cells with increased Hb F have a survival advantage.

The interaction of α-thalassemia with sickle cell anemia has been the subject of numerous studies. Sickle cell anemia patients with either α-thalassemia-1 or α-thalassemia-2 have reduced mean cell hemoglobin (MCH) and mean cell volume (MCV) values and slightly elevated Hb A_2. The coexistence of α-thalassemia and Hb S heterozygosity can have a marked effect in the level of Hb S. It is still not clear whether sickle cell anemia patients who may also have heterozygosity for α-thalassemia-1 or α-thalassemia-2, because they have less mean cell Hb S, are less severely affected than persons with *SS* condition alone. Different forms of Hb S β-thalassemia may result from the interaction of Hb S gene with either β^0- or β^+-thalassemia. The clinical course of sickle cell thalassemia may range from one extreme in which the condition is indistinguishable from sickle cell anemia to a disorder that is completely symptomless.

The combination of Hb S and Hb C, i.e., a heterozygous state for the two abnormal hemoglobins, results in hemoglobin SC disease. Likewise, the combination of Hb S and Hb D results in Hb SD disease. In Hb SC disease, the anemia is mild, and indeed the hemoglobin level may be normal. Vascular complications arise in these patients not so much from anemia but from increased blood viscosity.

Before antisickling agents can be developed, the mechanism of sickling has to be elucidated with certainty. In fact, significant information with regard to the orientation of individual macromolecules within the filaments that constitute the fiber has been gained by electron microscopy and image reconstruction and by x-ray diffraction measurements. At present, the concept of 14-strand arrangement (ten outer filaments surrounding four inner ones) occurring in the majority of the aggregated Hb S molecules in a sickled erythrocyte seems to be generally acceptable. The points of contact between Hb molecule in the fiber were also delineated by electron microscopic and x-ray work and from sickling tendencies of double mutants. Approaches to specific antisickling therapies at the molecular, the cellular, and the individual levels are (a) inhibition of Hb S contacts in gel by noncovalent and covalent reagents, (b) decrease in deoxy-Hb S concentration by increasing oxygen affinity and decreasing total Hb S concentration, (c) cell sickling inhibitors or membrane modifiers, and (d) inhibitors of microvascular entrapment. Aliphatic and aromatic aldehydes (Schiff-base adducts) are of particular interest as they are potential gelation inhibitors by inhibiting Hb S contacts in gel or by increasing the oxygen affinity (decreasing deoxy-Hb S concentration).

C. The Thalassemias

The thalassemias are an extremely diverse group of disorders of hemoglobin synthesis, with reduction or even complete absence in the output of specific globin chains (5). The more we know about the genetic basis of the various forms of the thalassemias, the more complex the classification of the thalassemias is becoming. In general, thalassemias may be classified as α-thalassemia, β-thalassemia, δβ-thalassemia, δ-thalassemia, and γδβ-thalassemia. α-Thalassemia can be due to α-thalassemia-1, α-thalassemia-2, or inefficient synthesis of some α chain variants. β-Thalassemia is of two major types, namely, β^0-thalassemia and β^+-thalassemia, although several subclassifications of each of these also exist.

Two types of α-thalassemia, the severe form or α-thalassemia-1 and a mild form or α-thalassemia-2 have been recognized during early work. In many cases, α-thalassemia-1 results from the deletion of two α-globin genes, while α-thalassemia-2 results from the loss of one gene. Thus, the heterozygous genotypes for these conditions are written --/αα and -α/αα and haplotypes as -- and -α, respectively. An individual who is homozygous for α-thalassemia-2 (-α/-α) will have two active α-globin genes and the same phenotype as an individual heterozygous for α-thalassemia-1. Phenotype similar to α-thalassemia-1 is seen with Hb Constant Spring. Heterozygosity for both α-thalassemia-1 and α-thalassemia-2 (--/-α) results in Hb H (β_4) disease. The outcome of complete suppression of the α-chain synthesis is hemoglobin Bart's (γ_4) hydrops fetalis syndrome. The hemoglobin of such a child consists of only Hb H, Hb Bart's, and Hb Portland 1. The genetic basis for this condition is the homozygosity for α-thalassemia-1 (--/--). Newborns with α-thalassemia-1 have 5-10% Hb Bart's, low MCH, and low MCV. Newborns with α-thalassemia-2, on the other hand, have 0-2% Hb Bart's with minimal hematological changes. Recent gene mapping analysis has shown that there are a series of molecular defects that can give rise to both α-thalassemia-1 and -2 phenotypes. One also has to reckon with nondeletion α-thalassemia and dysfunctional α-thalassemia.

β-Thalassemia can be subdivided into two main classes, namely, β^+-thalassemia and β^0-thalassemia. Homozygosity for these conditions is commonly referred to as Cooley's anemia or thalassemia major. In 1925, Cooley and Lee described this condition. Phenotypically, "β^+" denotes synthesis of some β chains, although there is significant suppression, and "β^0" denotes total absence of the β-chain production. Heterozygotes for β^+-thalassemia or β^0-thalassemia (thalassemia minor) have elevated Hb A_2 (3.5-7.2%) and slight elevation of Hb F accompanied by variable anemia. Homozygosity for β^+-thalassemia is associated with 20-80% Hb F, variable Hb A_2, and free α chains. In β^0-

thalassemia homozygotes, the entire hemoglobin is fetal type with no Hb A_2 and Hb A. Patients with these conditions have severely affected anemia requiring rather frequent blood transfusion. Several variations of the β^0-thalassemia and β^+-thalassemia are known to exist. Some are defined at the molecular level and some at the phenotypic level only. On the basis of clinical severity, β^+-thalassemia is of the severe Mediterranean type and of the mild Negro type. There is also the so-called "silent" β-thalassemia with normal Hb A_2. $\delta\beta$-Thalassemia is of ${}^G\gamma{}^A\gamma$ $(\delta\beta)^0$-thalassemia, ${}^G\gamma$ $(\delta\beta)^0$-thalassemia, and Hb Lepore $(\delta\beta)^+$-thalassemia types. A patient with heterozygosity for β^0-thalassemia and for $(\delta\beta)^0$-thalassemia would have mild Cooley's anemia, with Hb F making up the total hemoglobin except a trace amount of Hb A_2.

D. Hereditary Persistence of Fetal Hemoglobin

Hereditary persistence of fetal hemoglobin (HPFH) represents a group of conditions characterized by persistence of fetal hemoglobin synthesis into adult life in the absence of significant hematological manifestations. This condition has much in common with $\delta\beta$- and β-thalassemia. In contrast to β^0-thalassemia, however, the fetal hemoglobin production in HPFH almost entirely compensates for the absence of adult hemoglobin. The relatively homogeneous distribution of Hb F throughout the red cells has been used to disinguish the condition from disorders, such as thalassemia and sickle cell anemia, where Hb F is more or less heterogeneously distributed among red cells. The structural analysis of Hb F from individuals with HPFH allowed a further classification on the basis of Hb F types, i.e., ${}^G\gamma{}^A\gamma$ HPFH, ${}^G\gamma$ HPFH, and ${}^A\gamma$ HPFH. In the heterozygous state, this condition can coexist with variants Hb S, Hb C, Hb E, etc., and with β-thalassemia and δ-thalassemia. A unique type of HPFH, where the Hb F is heterogenously distributed among the red cells, i.e., "heterocellular HPFH" as opposed to "pancellular HPFH," also has been described.

LIST OF ABBREVIATIONS

ALA	δ-aminolevulinic acid
DABITC	4-N, N-dimethylaminoazobenzene-4′-isothiocyanate
2,3-DPG	2,3-diphosphoglycerate
Hb	hemoglobin
HPFH	hereditary persistence of hemoglobin
PITC	phenylisothiocyanate

REFERENCES

1. H. Lehman and R. G. Huntsman, *Man's Hemoglobins,* J. B. Lippincott, Co., Philadelphia (1973).
2. S. Granick and R. D. Levere, *Prog. Hematol., 4:* 1 (1964).
3. H. F. Bunn, B. G. Forget, and H. M. Ranney, *Human Hemoglobins,* Sanders, Philadelphia (1977).
4. T. H. J. Huisman and J. H. P. Jonxis, *The Hemoglobinopathies: Techniques of Identification,* Marcel Dekker, New York (1971).
5. D. J. Weatherall and J. B. Clegg, *The Thalassemia Syndrome,* Blackwell Scientific Publication, London (1981).
6. E. Antonini and M. Brunori, *Hemoglobin and Myoglobin in Their Reactions with Ligands,* North-Holland, Amsterdam (1971).
7. C. D. Coryell and L. Pauling, *J. Biol. Chem., 132:* 769 (1940).
8. A. F. Cullis, H. Mruihead, M. F. Perutz, M. G. Rossman, and A. C. T. North, *Proc. Roy. Soc., A265:* 161 (1962).
9. M. F. Perutz, *Sci. Am., 211*(11): 64 (1964).
10. M. F. Perutz, *Nature* (*London*), *228*: 726 (1970).
11. E. A. Rachmilewitz, *Sem. Hemat., 21:* 441 (1974).
12. W. A. Schroeder, *The Primary Structure of Proteins,* Harper and Row, New York (1968).
13. T. Liu, A. Schecter, R. Heinrikson, and P. Condliffe, *Chemical Synthesis and Sequencing of Peptides and Proteins,* Elsevier/North-Holland, Amsterdam (1980).
14. R. L. Lundblad and C. M. Noyes, *Chemical Reagents for Protein Modification,* CRC Press, Boca Raton, Florida (1984).
15. M. F. Perutz, H. Muirhead, J. M. Cox, and L. C. G. Croaman, *Nature* (*London*), *219:* 131 (1968).
16. W. Bolton and M. F. Perutz, *Nature* (*London*), *228:* 551 (1970).
17. M. F. Perutz and H. Lehman, *Nature* (*London*), *219:* 902 (1968).
18. C. Bohr, K. Hasselbalch, and A. Krogh, *Skandinav, Arch. Physiol., 16:* 402 (1904).
19. A. V. Hill, *J. Physiol., 40:* 4P (1910).
20. G. S. Adair, *J. Biol. Chem., 63:* 529 (1925).
21. F. S. W. Roughton, A. B. Otis, and R. L. S. Lyster, *Proc. Roy. Soc., B144:* 29 (1955).
22. Q. H. Gibson and F. J. W. Roughton, *Proc. Roy. Soc., B146:* 206 (1957).
23. J. Christiansen, C. G. Doublas, and J. S. Haldane, *J. Physiol., 48:* 224 (1914).
24. L. J. Henderson, *J. Biol. Chem., 41:* 401 (1920).
25. J. Wyman, *Advan. Prot. Chem., 4:* 407 (1948).

26. L. Rossi-Bernardi and F. J. W. Roughton, *J. Biol. Chem., 242:* 784 (1967).
27. A. Chanutin and R. R. Churnish, *Arch. Biochem. Biophys., 121:* 96 (1967).
28. R. Benesch and R. E. Benesch, *Nature* (*London*), *221:* 618 (1969).
29. R. Benesch, R. E. Benesch, and Y. Enoki, *Proc. Natl. Acad. Sci., USA, 61:* 1102 (1968).
30. R. Benesch, R. E. Benesch, and C. I. Yu, *Proc. Natl. Acad. Sci., USA, 159:* 526 (1968).

3

Structure, Function, and Biosynthesis of Glycosylated Hemoglobins

I. STRUCTURAL ASPECTS

A. Chromatographic Purification of Glycosylated Hemoglobins

In adults and children above the age of 6 months, Hb A ($\alpha_2\beta_2$) constitutes about 97% and HbA$_2$ ($\alpha_2\delta_2$) and Hb F constitutes ($\alpha_2\gamma_2$) about 2.5 and 0.5%, respectively, of the total hemoglobin (Hb). The synthesis of these hemoglobins are genetically controlled, the α, β, δ, and γ chains being coded by separate genes. About 6% of the total Hb A contains a group of minor hemoglobins termed Hb A_I having electrophoretic and chromatographic properties different from the major component, namely, Hb A_o (Hb A_{II} according to old literature). These minor hemoglobins were initially separated by Amberlite IRC-50 chromatography and termed Hb A_{Ia}, Hb A_{Ib}, Hb A_{Ic}, Hb A_{Id}, and Hb A_{Ie} according to the order in which they were eluted from Amberlite IRC-50 columns (1,2) (Fig. 3.1). The chromatographic separations were achieved by Schroeder and co-workers (1,2) by applying 50 to 60 mg of hemoglobin onto 1 X 35 cm columns of the IRC-50 resin and developing with a stepwise gradient of sodium phosphate. The columns were developed at 5-6°C first

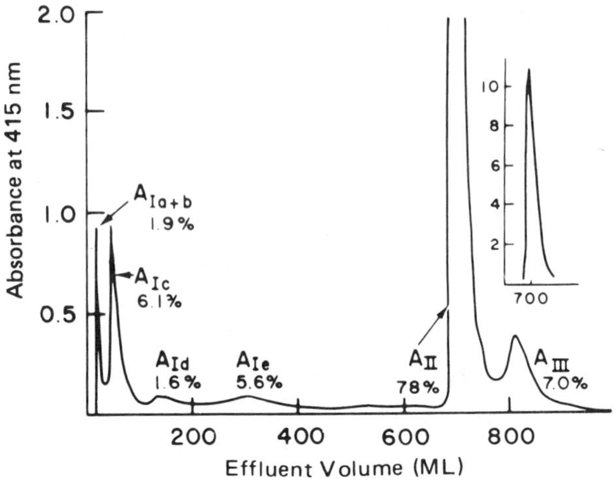

Figure 3.1 The separation of the various hemoglobin components from a hemolysate of normal red blood cells by Amberlite IRC-50 chromatography. Reproduced from Schnek and Schroeder (2) by permission of the American Chemical Society.

and then at room temperature. By this approach, complete separation of Hb A_{Ia} and Hb A_{Ib} was not accomplished. As the conditions of the chromatography and the gradient were modified, more and more heterogeneity of the minor components were revealed. For instance, by utilizing Bio-Rex 70 resin and a linear sodium chloride gradient at 4°C (3), Hb A_{Ia} was resolved into two components termed Hb A_{Ia1} and Hb A_{Ia2}. Surprisingly, Hb A_{Id} and Hb A_{Ie} were not seen in those chromatograms. With this chromatographic system, the percentages of Hb A_{Ia1}, Hb A_{Ia2}, Hb A_{Ib}, and Hb A_{Ic} in normal adults were about 0.2, 0.2, 0.5, and 3.5%, respectively. Depending upon the chromatographic procedure, the Hb A_{Ia1} could be contaminated with nonheme proteins coeluting with this fraction. Further improvement of the Bio-Rex 70 chromatographic procedure, using a slowly increasing sodium phosphate gradient at 4°C, has enabled us to separate up to nine minor Hb components from normal and diabetic adults (Fig. 3.2) (4). Nonheme proteins were eluted first, followed by Hb components A_{Ia1}, A_{Ia2}, A_{Ib1}, A_{Ib2}, A_{Ib3}, A_{Ic}, A_{Id1}, A_{Id2}, and A_{Id3}. All these minor hemoglobin components, except A_{Ia1}, A_{Ia2}, and A_{Ib1}, were significantly increased in pateints with diabetes (Table 3.1). With a 2 × 25 cm column of Bio-Rex 70, 200-300 mg of Hb could be processed. Separation of the various minor Hbs was also achieved in our

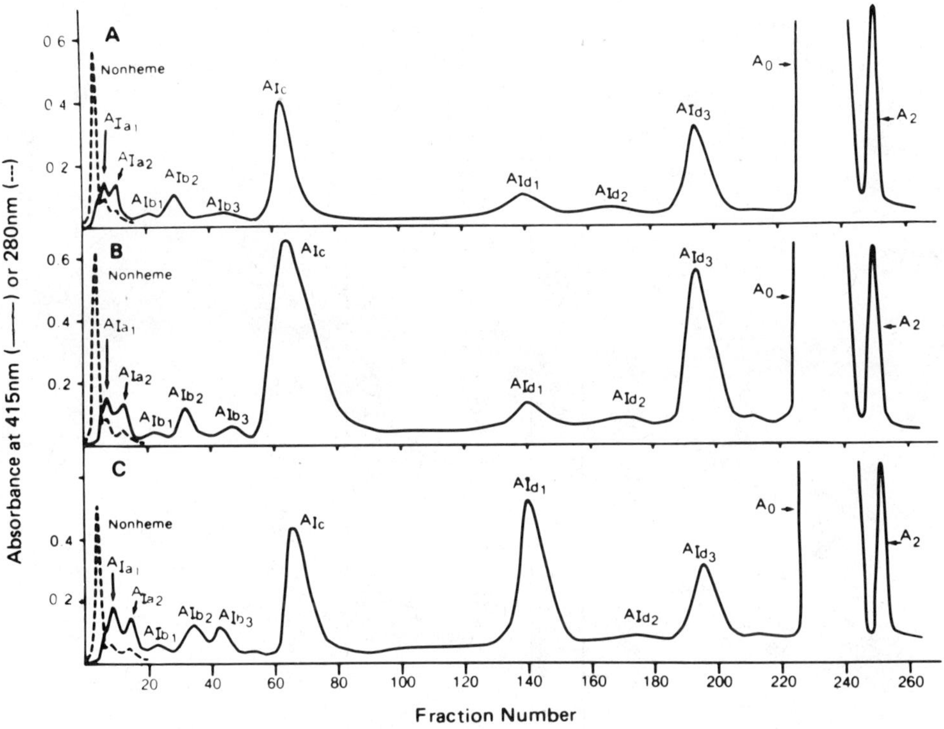

Figure 3.2 Bio-Rex 70 chromatographic separation of the minor hemoglobins in red cell hemolysates of (A) a normal adult, (B) a patient with insulin-dependent diabetes mellitus, and (C) a normal adult after incubation with 7 mM oxidized glutathione. About 250 mg was applied to a 3 X 30 cm column and developed at 4°C with a flow rate of 24 ml/hr and 8 ml fractions were collected. A sodium phosphate gradient was applied with Developers 6, 8, and 10 (see Chap. 4). From Abraham et al. (4) by permission of the Elsevier Biomedical Press.

laboratory by a newly introduced high-pressure liquid chromatographic (HPLC) procedure, which utilized Synchropak CM 300 cation exchange column with Bis-Tris developers and linear sodium acetate gradient (5,6) (Fig. 3.3). However, since only 200-300 μg Hb were separated at a time, the quantities of the components recovered were too small for further studies.

Table 3.1 Percentages of Minor Hemoglobin Components in Normal Adults (n=10) and in Patients with Insulin-Dependent Diabetes Mellitus (n=11)[a]

Samples	A_{Ia1}	A_{Ia2}	A_{Ib1}	A_{Ib2}	A_{Ib3}	A_{Ic}	A_{Id1}	A_{Id2}	A_{Id3}	$A_o + A_2$
Normals	0.37	0.27	0.25	0.59	0.36	5.03	0.35	0.60	1.93	90.01
	±0.03	±0.03	±0.05	±0.09	±0.12	±0.69	±0.11	±0.23	±0.19	±1.01
Diabetics	0.37	0.37	0.34	1.05	0.65	9.04	0.64	1.15	3.22	84.49
	±0.06	±0.13	±0.15	±0.46	±0.20	±2.26	±0.24	±0.22	±0.60	±3.18

[a]Results are given as the mean ± standard deviation.
Source: From Abraham et al. (4) by permission of the Elsevier Biomedical Press.

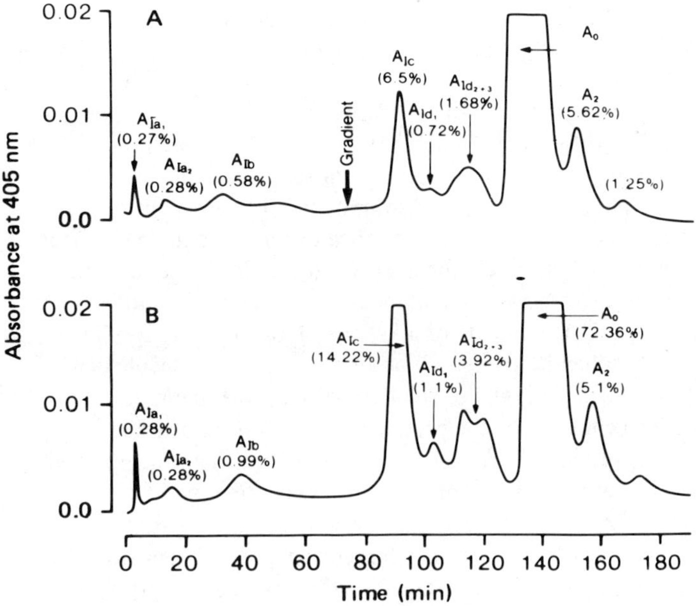

Figure 3.3 Separation of the various minor hemoglobin components in a normal adult (A) and in a diabetic (B) by high-pressure liquid chromatography (HPLC) with a Synchropak CM 300 cation exchange column. Three hundred micrograms of hemoglobin (dialyzed against the starting buffer) were applied to the column and developed with Bis-Tris developers and a linear sodium acetate gradient applied after an initial isocratic step. A flow rate of 1 ml/min was maintained. The HPLC system used was a Beckman Model 330 with 110A pumps, Model 160 detector, Model 421 microprocessor-controller. Absorbances at 405 nm were traced and integrated with a Hewlett-Packard Model 3390A recorder-integrator (see Chap. 4 for further details).

B. Structure of Hb A_{Ic}

Most of the attention in the structural characterization was given to Hb A_{Ic}, which constitutes the major portion of the total glycosylated hemoglobins. Moreover, the major obstacle in analyzing these hemoglobins was that the other minor hemoglobins were present in fairly small amounts. The earlier work of Holmquist and Schroeder (7) was the key in determining the structural difference between Hb A_o and Hb A_{Ic}. Large amunts of Hb A_{Ic} were purified from large (10 × 100 cm) Bio-Rex 70 columns. Up to 2 g of Hb A_{Ic} could be isolated from 1 pint of blood. β_{Ic} Chains were separated from Hb A_{Ic} and β_o chains from Hb A_o after removal of the heme. Tryptic peptides were prepared and separated on cation exchange or anion exchange columns; βT-1, βIc T-1, and sodium borohydride ($NaBH_4$)-reduced βIc T-1 were prepared and further treated with papain. Thus Val-His, R-Val-His, and reduced R-Val-His peptides were prepared. The amino acid composition of each peptide was determined by amino acid analysis, the sequence by the Edman degradation, and the N-terminal analysis by the Sanger's procedure. It was concluded from these studies that Hb A_{Ic} is the condensation product (a Schiff base) of 1 molecule of Hb A_o and 1 molecule of a ketone or an aldehyde R=O (the present concept is 2 molecules of ketone or aldehyde for 1 molecule of Hb A_o). The point of linkage of R=O to the hemoglobin was the N terminus of the β chains. Strong evidence for the presence of a Schiff-base adduct was also found. The pK_a of this Schiff base was 6.64. Other than this, no difference has been found between the primary structure of the α and β chains of Hb A_o and Hb A_{Ic}. The keto or aldehyde group had a molecular weight of approximately 280. Carbohydrate was excluded as a possible identity for the R=O group, but long-chain aromatic aldehyde or ketone was strongly suggested. In Hb A_{Ic}, only one of the β chain was originally thought to have undergone Schiff-base formation. Later studies by Bookchin and Gallop (8) established that a hexose is linked to the amino terminus of both β chains of Hb A_{Ic}. They examined the structure of the blocking group by mass spectrometry. Tritiated *N*-alkylated valine was prepared by acid hydrolysis of Hb A_{Ic} after reducing the linkage with NaB^3H_4. Mass spectral analysis was possible after reacting the tritiated product with acetic anhydride. The mass spectrum of the acetylated derivative was consistent with *N*-1-(1-deoxyhexitol)- or *N*-1-(1-galactitol)valine. Thus, it was established that a simple sugar rather than a long-chain aldehyde or a ketone is attached to each of the β chains in Hb A_{Ic}.

It is rather puzzling that although glucose is considered to be the most logical substrate in the glycosylation reaction, the N terminus is a *N*-1-(deoxygalactitol)valine. Thus, it is possible that a rearrangement has taken place after the initial reaction, namely, the Schiff-base formation. When Hb A_{Ic} was subjected to mild acid hydrolysis, reducing sugars were formed (9). In fact, glucose and mannose present in a 3:1 ratio accounted for nearly all the reducing sugars. The appearance of mannose in the hydrolysate cannot be explained, since red cells contain little or no mannose. Just as in Maillard browning reaction, in red cells, glucose reacts initially with the amino-terminal groups of the β chain to form an aldimine linkage, which subsequently undergoes Amadori rearrangement to form a more stable ketoamine linkage (see Fig. 1.1). The evidence for this was obtained as follows: When Hb A_{Ic} was treated with [^{3}H] $NaBH_4$ and then with sodium periodate, nearly all the radioactivity was recovered as [^{3}H] formic acid (9). If the major portion of the sugar was linked to the protein through a Schiff base, most of the radioactivity should have been recovered as [^{3}H] formaldehyde. This observation suggested that the second carbon atom rather than the first was reduced. Additional evidence was gathered to support Amadori rearrangement as an integral step even in in vivo glycosylation reactions. Such evidence came from the proton magnetic resonance spectroscopic and thin-layer chromatographic and gas-liquid chromatographic analyses of β-chain N-terminal peptides, Val-His and R-Val-His, and synthetic model compounds (10). In addition, model reactions showed that glucose and mannose reacted with valine of synthetic Val-His under mild conditions to form an adduct that, upon $NaBH_4$ reduction, yielded glucitol- and mannitol-valines in both cases. The simple fact that 5-hydroxymethylfurfural (5-HMF) can be formed by heating Hb A_{Ic} with mild oxalic acid is consistent with the ketoamine linkage (see Fig. 4.29) (11).

C. Structure of Hb A_{Ia1} and Hb A_{Ia2}

Several approaches were adopted for elucidation of the structure of Hb A_{Ia1} and Hb A_{Ia2}. Most of the evidence was rather indirect and circumstantial. The fact that Hb A_{Ia1} migrated faster than Hb A_{Ia2} and that Hb A_{Ia2} was faster than Hb A_{Ic} clearly indicated that there is a clear-cut difference in the net charges on these proteins, Hb A_{Ia1} being the most negatively charged (3). One of the approaches used was to synthesize these minor hemoglobins by cell-free glycosylation of Hb A_o with two radiolabeled phosphorylated glycolytic intermediates, namely, fructose 1,6-diphosphate (FDP) and glucose 6-phosphate (G6P) (3,12,13). When chromatographically purified Hb A_o was incubated with [^{14}C] FDP and [^{14}C] G6P, radioactivity peaks were seen primarily associated with Hb F_{Ia1} and Hb F_{Ia2} zones, respectively. About 95% of the radioactivity was bound to the β-chain NH_2-terminal amino acids. Both of these intermediates reacted with Hb A_o about 20-fold faster than glucose. Evidence indicated that these two compounds serve as affinity labels through phosphate groups, while the aldehyde groups form covalent Schiff-base linkages. The ^{32}P nuclear magnetic resonance spectrum of synthetic G6P-hemoglobin was also identical to that of Hb A_{Ia2}.

Analysis of the various Hb components for protein-bound ketoamine and

Table 3.2 Results of the Colorimetric Assay (TBA Assay) for Ketoamine and Phosphate Analysis of Hemoglobin Components

Hb component	TBA assay (A_{443})	Phosphate content (mol P/$\alpha\beta$ dimer)
Hb A_{Ia1}	0.105	1.9
Hb A_{Ia2}	0.114	1.2
Hb A_{Ib1}	0.153	1.1
Hb A_{Ib2}	0.128	0.2
Hb A_{Ib3}	0.275	0.8
Hb A_{Ic}	0.380	0.1
Hb A_{Id1}	0.102	0.5
Hb A_{Id2}	0.089	0.1
Hb A_{Id3}	0.083	0
Hb A_o	0.043	0

Source: From Abraham et al. (4) by permission of the Elsevier Biomedical Press.

phosphate was another way of confirming the conclusion made by in vitro glycosylation experiments. According to Flückiger and Winterhalter (11), when glycosylated components were treated with dilute oxalic acid at 100°C, the protein-bound ketoamine was released as 5-HMF. This product when complexed with thiobarbituric acid (TBA) produced a characteristic spectrum with λ_{max} of 443 nm. This observation has become the basis for the colorimetric assay (TBA assay) for protein-bound ketoamine, although the original methodology has undergone substantial refinement. Table 3.2 gives the results of TBA assay of a variety of Hb components (3,4). On the basis of this assay, Hb A_{Ic} contains most of the ketoamine and Hb A_{Ia1} and Hb A_{Ia2} contain only one-third of the ketoamine that is present in Hb A_{Ic}. It is difficult to understand this unless we believe that Hb A_{Ia1} and Hb A_{Ia2} are relatively impure or that the phosphorylated sugars are not efficiently converted to 5-HMF. It is likely that the ketoamine linkage of these Hbs are relatively stable. If indeed Hb A_{Ia1} contains 2 mol of FDP and Hb A_{Ia2} contains 1 mol of G6P per mole of Hb, on analysis of the Hb-bound phosphate, one expects to see 4 and 2 mol of phosphorus per tetramer of hemoglobin. In fact, this was confirmed by more than one laboratory (3,4) (Table 3.2). To determine this, the unbound phosphate was removed by gel filtration, the protein was precipitated with trichloroacetic and digested with sulfuric acid, and the color was developed by the ammonium molybdate reagent. These studies strongly indicated that Hb A_{Ia1} and Hb A_{Ia2} are formed by reaction of the NH_2-terminal groups of both β chains of Hb A_o with FDP and G6P, respectively. However, absolute proof for the nature of the modification in these minor hemoglobins is still lacking.

D. Structure of Hb A_{Ib}

Hemoglobin A_{Ib} is one of the least characterized of all the minor hemoglobins. The presence of at least three types of Hb A_{Ib} (A_{Ib1}, A_{Ib2}, and A_{Ib3}) has been recognized (Fig. 3.2) (4). The percentages of Hb A_{Ib1}, Hb A_{Ib2}, and Hb A_{Ib3} in normal adults are 0.25, 0.59, and 0.36%, respectively, whereas insulin-dependent diabetic patients have 0.34, 1.05, and 0.65%, respectively (Table 3.1). All the three Hb A_{Ib} components contain significant amounts of ketoamine, Hb A_{Ib3} containing the largest amount (Table 3.2). No significant amounts of Hb-bound organic phosphate are present in Hb A_{Ib1} and Hb A_{Ib2}, whereas Hb A_{Ib3} contains about 1.6 mol of phosphate per tetramer of Hb. These results are inconclusive, and the nature of the modification in these hemoglobins are still unknown. Two other studies have shed some light into the structural heterogeneity of Hb A_{Ib} (separated as one component). The early work of Holmquist and Schroeder (7) showed Hb A_{Ib} to be a glycosylated component modified at the NH_2 terminus of the β chain. According to Krishnamoorthy et al. (14), the modification is on the β chain but not at the NH_2 terminus. These authors have purified Hb A_{Ib} by polyacrylamide gel electrofocusing and attempted to determine its structure and function. Structural and functional heterogeneities observed were consistent with a hybrid structure of $\alpha_2\beta^A\beta^X$ having only one of its β chains chemically modified. This modification seems to perturb the quaternary structure of the Hb molecule, and this perturbation may be predominate at lower pH values. At pH 6.5 or below, dissociation and reassociation of Hb A_{Ib} may be leading to the formation of the hybrid molecule. In fact, such a scheme explains some of the functional, structural, and chromatographic heterogeneities observed at pH 6.5. It has been hypothesized that the chemical modification in Hb A_{Ib} is deamidation of a β-chain glutamine or asparagine (14). However, the fact that ketoamine is present in this component(s) cannot be reconciled with this concept. Until demonstrated otherwise, Hb A_{Ib} is considered a glycosylated component(s).

E. Structure of Hb A_{Id}

About 25 years ago, the presence of Hb A_{Id} in adult red cell hemolysate was demonstrated by Schroeder and his associates (1,2) by performing Amberlite IRC-50 chromatography. This component was found to constitute about 1.6% of the total Hb in normal adults. The probability of detecting and quantifying always depended on the chromatographic method and the storage conditions of the blood samples. Dozy and Huisman (15) found increased formation of Hb A_{Id} during prolonged storage of red cell hemolysate stored undialyzed or in the presence of glutathione. It is believed that during this period, glutathione (GSH) is subjected to oxidation to form oxidized glutathione (GSSG). Oxidized glutathione and the free –SH groups of the Hb molecule undergo disulfide interchange to form HbSSG. Apparently β93 cysteine of both β chains undergo this modification. As compared to Hb A_o, this modified Hb has increased mobility on electrophoresis at an alkaline pH and on cation exchange columns and decreased mobility on DEAE-cellulose columns.

Hemoglobin A_{Id} normally migrates with the rest of the Hb A_{Is} on alkaline electrophoresis. A linear sodium phosphate gradient system is needed to separate it from Hb A_o during Bio-Rex 70 cation exchange chromatography. When a simple two-step phosphate gradient was applied according to Trivelli et al. (16), Hb A_{Id} seemed to be eluted with Hb A_o (Fig. 3.4 and see Fig. 4.4). Application of an improved Bio-Rex 70 chromatographic method has enabled us to further fractionate Hb A_{Id} into three different minor Hbs, termed A_{Id1}, A_{Id2}, and A_{Id3} (Fig. 3.2 and Table 3.1) (4). The percentages of Hb A_{Id1}, A_{Id2}, and A_{Id3} in normal adults were about 0.35, 0.6, and 1.93%, respectively; these levels were increased about twofold in diabetic patients. All the three Hb components contained Hb-bound ketoamine, although not as much as in Hb A_{Ic} (Table 3.2). Only trace amounts of phosphate were seen in these components, except in Hb A_{Id1}, which contained 0.5 mol phosphate per Hb dimer. When a red cell hemolysate was incubated with GSSG, significant increase in the Hb A_{Id1} fraction was observed, indicating that the component formed by the disulfide interchange reaction will migrate in the position of Hb A_{Id1}. Since Hb A_{Id1} also contains ketoamine, heterogeneity seems to exist even in this component that is normally present in fairly small amounts in a freshly prepared hemolysate. The identity of Hb A_{Id2} is not established, although it seems to be a glycosylated component. Hemoglobin A_{Id3} is present in relatively large amounts, next only to Hb A_{Ic}, in normal and diabetic samples (1.9 and 3.2%, respectively). This fraction has been subjected to extensive structural and functional studies (4). On globin chain electrophoresis in the presence of 6 M urea and β-mercaptoethanol at pH 8.6,

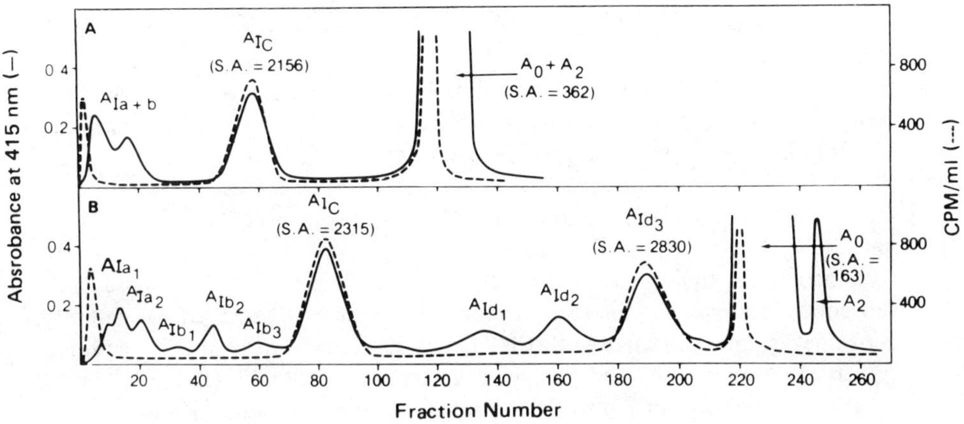

Figure 3.4 Separation of the hemoglobins by Bio-Rex 70 chromatography in a red cell hemolysate after incubation with [^{14}C]glucose. (A) Chromatography according to a "stepwise-elution" system of Trivelli et al. (16). (B) Chromatography according to a gradient-elution system of Abraham et al. (4). The specific activity (S.A.) of each hemoglobin component (cpm/1.0 absorbance) is also given. From Abraham et al. (4) by permission of the Elsevier Biomedical Press.

the cathodal mobility of the α chains of Hb A_{Id3} was slower than that of the normal α chains of Hb A_o. As expected, the anodal mobility of the β chains of Hb A_{Ic} was significantly greater than that of the β chains of Hb A_o. This strongly indicates that the α chain of Hb A_{Id3} is modified. However, it is surprising that the ketaomine content is significantly lower than in Hb A_{Ic}, unless inadequate release of 5-HMF from the α-chain NH_2-terminus-bound ketoamine is the reason for this (Table 3.2). It should be pointed out here that Bunn and his co-workers (17,18) confirmed the existence of a glycosylated component whose α-chain amino-terminal amino acids are modified. However, they were not able to separate this component by any chromatographic means available to them.

In the early studies of Clegg and Schroeder (1), a broad peak eluted after Hb A_{Id} was termed Hb A_{Ie}; however, its identity is not known. It is very likely that the Hb A_{Ie} represents one of the subfractions of Hb A_{Id} observed in later studies (4).

F. Other Types of Glycosylated Hemoglobins

We have already discussed a variety of glycosylated hemoglobins that are formed by attachment of glucose or phosphorylated intermediates at the NH_2-terminal amino acids of the β chains or the α chains. Moreover, glycosylation can occur at the ϵ-amino groups of lysine residues, despite their relatively high pK_a. The indication that extra sites are contributing to glycosylation came from in vitro glycosylation studies with ^{14}C-labeled glucose, G6P, and FDP (11,17-21,4). As early as 1976, Flückiger and Winterhalter (11), while performing in vitro glycosylation of Hb A_o by incubating with [^{14}C]glucose and subsequently separating the Hbs on Bio-Rex 70 columns, observed two radioactive peaks, one associated with Hb A_{Ic} and the other, unexpectedly, with Hb A_o. Incubation with ^{14}C-labeled glucose, G6P, and FDP with Hb F_o and Hb S_o also showed, in addition to the expected radioactivity under the appropriate minor Hb zones, large peaks of radioactivity at the leading edge of the major Hb zones (4,17-21). When Hb A_o was incubated with [^{14}C]glucose, a radioactivity peak matched the Hb A_{Ic} peak and another radioactivity peak appeared at the leading edge of Hb A_o (Fig. 3.4) (4). Additional radioactivity was associated with the Hb A_{Id3} peak if the chromatographic conditions were favorable for its separation. When the globin chains were separated by CM-cellulose chromatography, only the β_{Ic} chains, and not the α chains, in Hb A_{Ic} contained any appreciable radioactivity (Fig. 3.5). Nearly equal shares of the label were associated with the α and β chains of the Hb A_o peak. Interestingly, again the radioactivity peaks appeared at the leading edges of the α- and β-chain protein peaks. The initial interpretation for the presence of radioactivity under the major Hb zones was that it was due to "nonspecific" binding of glucose to hemoglobin. This nonspecific binding was rather insignificant with the phosphorylated sugars. With these sugar derivatives, about 95% of the binding was directed toward the α-amino groups of the β chains, presumably through an affinity labeling involving negatively charged phosphate moieties.

The additional sites of glycosylation on both the α and β chains were identified primarily in Bunn's laboratory (17,18). Both in vivo and in vitro glycosylation sites have been studied. To identify the in vitro glycosylated sites, Hb A_o was incubated with [^{14}C]glucose. The glycosylated components formed were separated by a DE52 anion exchange chromatography utilizing potassium tetraborate buffer. In this method, after elution of the major Hb peak, the total glycosylated hemoglobin was stripped off the column and subsequently reduced with unlabeled $NaBH_4$. Glycosylated peptides were isolated from tryptic digests of this hemoglobin by a com-

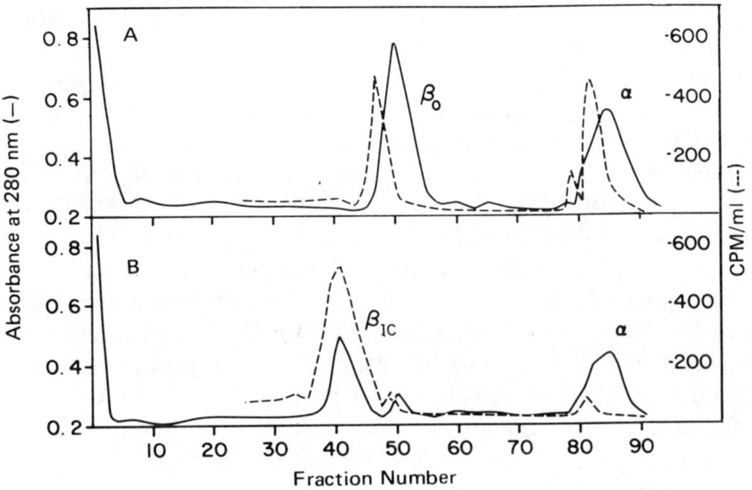

Figure 3.5 The separation by CM-cellulose chromatography of the chains of [^{14}C] glucose-labeled hemoglobins in the Hb A_0 (A) and Hb A_{Ic} (B) zones which have been isolated by Bio-Rex 70 chromatography (see Fig. 3.4).

bination of ion exchange chromatography and two-dimensional peptide mapping. Amino acid analysis of these peptides revealed the major sites of in vitro glycosylation (in order of prevalence) to be β-valine-1, α-lysine-16, β-lysine-66, β-lysine-17, α-valine-1, α-lysine-7, and β-lysine-120. For identification of the in vivo glycosylated sites, labeling of unincubated hemolysate with [^{3}H] borohydride was used. The major sites of in vivo glycosylation were (in order of prevalence) β-valine-1, β-lysine-66, α-lysine-61, β-lysine-17, and α-valine-1. α-Lysine-40, β-lysine-8, and β-lysine-144 were identified as the minor sites of in vivo glycosylation. Thus, significant differences between the sites of in vitro glycosylation and in vivo glycosylation were observed. However, one may want to modify the methodology for the identification of such sites by introducing affinity chromatographic steps (phenylboronate agarose and polyacrylamide) to purify glycosylated hemoglobins and peptides. This will simplify the identification of the glycosylation sites on various types of hemoglobins.

The available pK values for the various groups undergoing glycosylation do not explain the observed specificity with only the exception of the increased activity of the β NH_2 terminus. The pK_a of this group is close to

7 in contrast to 10 to 13 for the ϵ-amino groups. On the basis of such a large difference in the pK_a values, one would expect, at physiological conditions, over 100 times as many of the β NH_2 termini would be unprotonated as the ϵ-amino groups. The NH_2 terminus of the α chain has a pK_a between 7.6 and 7.8. However, it does not react as readily as some ϵ-NH_2 groups. Surprisingly, the glycosylated ϵ-NH_2 groups are not the ones with the lowest pK_a values; some of the most reactive groups have pK_a values greater than 11. The chromatographic behavior of the various glycosylated hemoglobins can be explained by the difference in the pK_a of the reactive groups. The ketoamine linkage at the amino groups does not remove the charge on these groups, but merely lowers their pK_a values. Amberlite IRC-50 or Bio-Rex 70 chromatography is normally performed at a pH near the pK_a of the β-chain amino terminus, and this condition obviously optimizes the separation of Hb A_{Ic}. However, the pK_a of the α-chain amino terminus is relatively high, and the change in pK_a due to glycosylation is slight. This explains why the separation of the hemoglobin glycosylated at the α-chain amino terminus is rather difficult and requires extremely shallow sodium phosphate gradient. The separation of the hemoglobins glycosylated at lysines from the major Hb A_o component is not possible by cation exchange chromatography because the chromatography is performed at least 4 units below the pK_a of the ϵ-amino groups.

II. GLYCOSYLATION AND HEMOGLOBIN FUNCTION

I have already discussed in an earlier chapter (Chap. 2) the role of 2,3-diphosphoglycerate (2,3-DPG), an intracellular organic phosphate in the regulation of oxygen transport. The negatively charged groups on this organic phosphate can form salt bridges with the positibely charged sites on the β chains at the central cavity of the Hb molecule, including the β-chain NH_2 terminus, which is one of the major sites of glycosylation. If this site is blocked, the binding of the 2,3-DPG molecule to Hb will be markedly reduced.

The functional properties of Hb A_{Ia1}, Hb A_{Ia2}, Hb A_{Ib}, Hb A_{Ic}, and Hb A_o have been determined in the presence and absence of organic phosphates (3,4,21,22). Oxygen equilibrium analyses were done in a tonometer with a recording spectrophotometer in the presence and absence of inositol hexaphosphate. In the absence of organic or inorganic phosphates, the oxygen affinities of Hb A_o, Hb A_{Ib}, and Hb A_{Ic} were high (P_{50} = 4.3-5.1 mm Hg in 0.1 M Bis-Tris, pH 7.0, at 20°C). On the other hand, under similar conditions, the oxygen affinities of Hb A_{Ia1} and Hb A_{Ia2} remained low (P_{50} = 14 and 8 mm Hg, respectively). Inositol hexaphosphate had a much

Table 3.3 Oxygen Affinities[a] and n Values of Minor Hb Components in the Presence and Absence of 2,3-Diphosphoglycerate (2,3-DPG)[a]

	- 2,3-DPG		+ 2 mM 2,3-DPG	
Hb component	P_{50} (mm Hg)	n value	P_{50} (mm Hg)	n value
Hb A_{Ia1}	14.3	1.6	14.5	1.8
Hb A_{Ia2}	8.8	1.6	9.2	1.7
Hb A_{Ib2}	5.5	2.2	6.8	2.1
Hb A_{Ic}	4.5	2.3	5.3	2.4
Hb A_{Id3}	3.0	2.2	8.0	2.5
Hb A_o	4.0	2.3	9.8	2.4

[a]P_{50} values were determined with a Hem-O-Scan at 37°C with Hb solutions of 6.4 g/dl in 0.1 M Bis-Tris-HCl, pH 7.0.

weaker effect on the oxygantion of the four glycosylated hemoglobins than of Hb A_o. Kinetic analysis of the carbon monoxide binding in the presence and absence of the same organic phosphate reflected the oxygen equilibria findings.

Table 3.3 gives the results obtained when the oxygen equilibrium analyses were done in a Hem-O-Scan in the presence or the absence of 2,3-DPG. 2,3-Diphosphoglycerate has very little effect on the oxygen affinities of Hb A_{Ia1}, Hb A_{Ia2}, Hb A_{Ib}, and Hb A_{Ic}. Hemoglobin A_{Id3} and Hb A_o, on the other hand, had significantly lower oxygen affinities in the presence of the organic phosphate (Fig. 3.6). This is not surprising because both of these hemoglobins have the β-chain amino terminus free for the binding of 2,3-DPG to occur. The amino-terminus modification of the α chains, as in Hb A_{Id3}, does not seem to affect the 2,3-DPG binding. This is not totally unexpected since Arnone's (23) x-ray diffraction studies have clearly shown the involvement of only β chains in 2,3-DPG binding.

It is easy to understand why Hb A_{Ic}, which has two sugar moieties covalently attached to the NH_2 termini of the β chains, has high oxygen affinity in the presence or absence of 2,3-DPG. Then, why do Hb A_{Ia1} and Hb A_{Ia2} have low affinities for ligands and also at the same time are insensitive to the presence of organic phosphates? It seems that the sugar phosphates that are covalently bound mimic the effect of free organic phosphates. Due to the covalent binding of FDP or G6P, it seems that the conformational equilibrium of the Hb molecule is already shifted to the tense or the deoxy conformation, thus lowering the oxygen affinity. The number of phosphate groups also

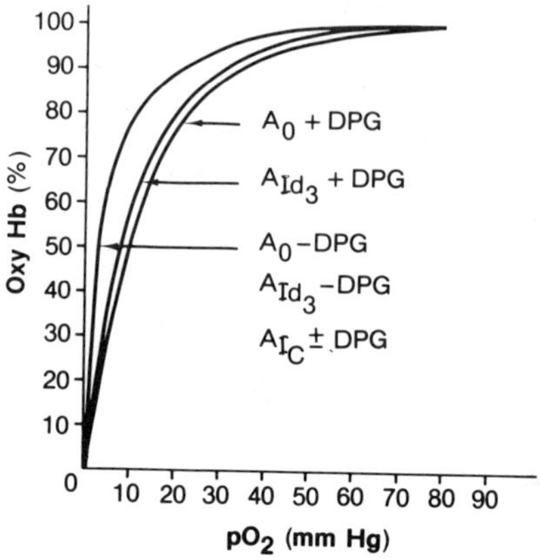

Figure 3.6 Oxyhemoglobin dissociation curves of Hb A_o, Hb A_{Ic}, and Hb A_{Id3} determined in 0.1 M Bis-Tris, pH 7.0 at 37°C in a Hem-O-Scan in the presence and absence of 2 mM 2,3-diphosphoglycerate (2,3-DPG). Reproduced from Abraham et al. (4) by permission of the Elsevier Biomedical Press.

seem to have direct bearing on the P_{50} values, as indicated by a difference in oxygen affinities between Hb A_{Ia1} and Hb_{Ia2}. All the minor Hbs except A_{Ic} exhibited a significant lowering of the Hill coefficient n. This may be due to the presence of multiple components of different functional characteristics or to α and β chain differences.

III. BIOSYNTHESIS OF GLYCOSYLATED HEMOGLOBINS

A. Glycosylation as a Posttranslational Modification

One can study the synthesis of hemoglobins in vitro in cell systems by following the incorporation of radiolabeled amino acids into the polypeptide portion or radiolabeled iron into the heme portion of the Hb molecule. Such studies were conducted by Bunn and his colleagues (24). The biosynthesis of glycosylated hemoglobins were studied in vitro by incubating reticulocytes with $[^3H]$leucine or bone marrow cells with ^{59}Fe-bound transferrin. If Hb A_{Ic} is formed from Hb A_o posttranslationally, i.e., after the completion of the Hb A_o synthesis, the specific activity of Hb A_{Ic} is expected to be lower than that of Hb A_o. In all experiments, the specific activity of Hb A_{Ic} was significantly lower than that of Hb A_o, suggesting that the formation of Hb A_{Ic} is a posttranslational event. Similar information was obtained by in vivo studies, where ^{59}Fe-bound transferrin was infused into individuals and the specific activities of the minor and the major Hbs were followed over a period of 100 days (24). Such experiments have shown that the specific activity of Hb A_o rose to a maximum in about one week, whereas the specific activities of Hb A_{Ic}, Hb A_{Ia}, and Hb A_{Ib} rose slowly, reaching that of Hb A_o in about 60 days. These results indicated that Hb A_{Ic} is slowly formed during the entire life span of the red cells. The data from these studies also best fit a slightly reversible model for Hb A_{Ic} synthesis. Studies by Koenig and Cerami (25) in nondiabetic (+/+) and diabetic (*db/db*) mice also were exceptionally useful. Adult diabetic mice had increased levels of a minor Hb that is similar in concentration and electrophoretic mobility to Hb A_{Ic} from human subjects. The concentration of this minor Hb was elevated only when the mice were diabetic. Moreover, when radiolabeled reticulocytes from normal or diabetic mice were injected into normal and diabetic mice, the rate of formation of the minor Hb was nearly three times faster when the donor cells circulated in a diabetic (*db/db*) recipient than when the cells circulated in a normal (+/+) recipient. Thus, the rate of synthesis of mouse Hb A_{Ic} was related to the environment in which the cells were circulating.

B. Glycosylation and Red Cell Age

The time dependence of Hb glycosylation is of biological significance. Glycosylation occurs slowly, continuously, and nearly irreversibly over the entire red cell life span. This means that the levels of glycosylated hemoglobins will be influenced by the red cell life span. Two observations are consistent with these conclusions. One is the finding of lower concentrations of glycosylated hemoglobin in hemolytic anemia (26), and the other is the finding of lower concentration of Hb A_{Ic} in young cells than in old cells (27-29). A curvilinear relationship between Hb A_I levels and red cell survival was demonstrated by Panzer et al. (26) in persons with hemolytic anemia with shorter red cell survival. Interestingly, after successful splenectomy of patients with hereditary spherocytosis, both red cell survival and Hb A_I levels increased. In nonhemolytic anemias, no decrease in Hb A_I was found. In patients with hemoglobinopathies with hemolytic episodes, for example, sickle cell anemia, glycosylated Hb levels were decreased considerably (27).

As early as 1960, Meyering et al. (28) have shown that glycosylated Hbs A_I, F_I, S_I, and E_I separated by CM-cellulose chromatography were present in relatively constant amounts in whole blood red cells, while their amounts were decreased in red cells of young mean cell age. These authors have fractionated the red cells into top, middle, and bottom portions by low-speed centrifugation. It was concluded from these studies that the above-mentioned glycosylated Hbs are formed in vivo as a result of changes in the corresponding major Hb, while the amounts of these minor fractions depend on the age of the circulating red blood cells.

Improved techniques for cell fractionation and for quantitation of glycosylated Hbs were used by Fitsgibbons et al. (29). They have used Dextran 40 isopycnic centrifugation to collect 10% youngest (lightest) and 10% oldest (heaviest) cell fractions. Hb A_{Ic} and Hb A_{Ia+b} were quantitated by Bio-Rex 70 chromatography for the youngest and the oldest cell fractions and for the unfractionated whole blood samples in normal and diabetic adults. Both normal and diabetic erythrocytes contained increased levels of the minor Hbs A_{Ia+b} and A_{Ic} in the old compared to the young cells. In normal subjects, the young cells contained 1.2% and the old cells contained 1.8% Hb A_{Ia+b}, whereas the corresponding values for the diabetics were 1.7 and 2.6%, respectively. Hemoglobin A_{Ic} increased from 3.1 to 6.0% in normals and from 5.1 to 10.1% in diabetics.

Red cell age-related changes in glycosylated hemoglobin levels were further investigated in our laboratory by Dextran 40 density gradient centrifugation for red cell fractionation (30) and by Bio-Rex 70 chromatography (for Hb A_{Ia+b} and Hb A_{Ic}), and affinity chromatography (for total glycosylated hemoglobin or GHb) for quantitation of glycosylated hemoglobins. The Dextran 40 technique for red cell fractionation utilized a discontinuous gradient made with Dextran 40 solutions of various densities and ultracentrifugation at 90,000 *g* (Fig. 3.7). Several discrete zones of red cells, separated according to their density (age), were collected and analyzed. Normal and diabetic adults, newborn babies, and patients with sickle cell anemia were used for these studies (27,31). Table 3.4 shows the hematologic characteristics of such red cell fractions of a normal adult and a newborn infant. The top cell layers contained the highest number of reticulocytes and had the highest mean cell volume (MCV). Mean cell volume decreased and MCHC (mean cell hemoglobin concentration) increased with an increase in red cell density (age). A linear increase in Hb A_{Ia+b} and Hb A_{Ic} in the normals and in a person with insulin-dependent diabetes mellitus (IDDM) was observed (Fig. 3.8). The total glycosylated hemoglobin (GHb) also showed a similar increase (Fig. 3.9). Although the absolute levels of GHb in the diabetic were significantly higher than in the normals, the increase in GHb with an increase

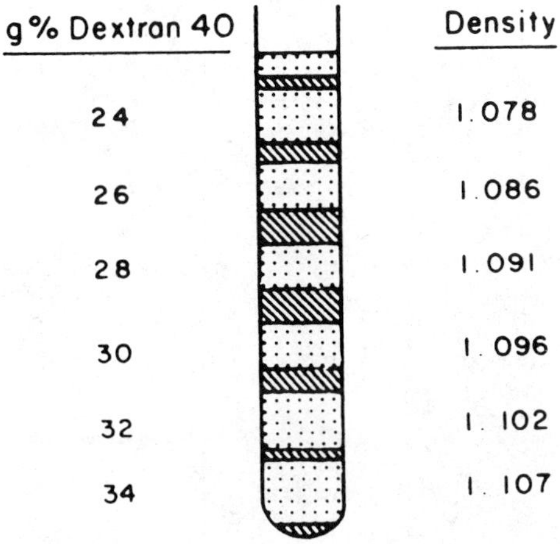

Figure 3.7 A schematic presentation of Dextran 40 discontinuous density gradient centrifugation; structure of the gradient and the position of the red cell zones. A discontinuous gradient is formed with Dextran 40 solutions (prepared in a standard medium plus deionized water) of 24 to 34 g/dl and densities of 1.078 to 1.107. Red cell suspension is layered over the gradient and centrifuged in an ultracentrifuge at 90,000 *g* for 90 min. Reproduced from Abraham et al. (30) by permission of the Academic Press, Inc.

in red cell density or age was nearly the same in both groups. The level of GHb and its increase with an increase in red cell density were significantly lower in newborn babies and in sickle cell anemia patients, reflecting reduced red cell survival in these two groups (Chap. 5). Thus, red cell age and diabetes are significant determinants of the concentration of glycosylated hemoglobins.

C. Kinetics of Nonenzymatic Glycosylation

Basically, three rate constants will be discussed: the first for the formation of the aldimine Schiff base (pre-A_{Ic}) by the condensation of free glucose with β-chain NH_2-terminal groups of Hb A_o (k_1), and the second is for the dissociation of the Schiff base to free glucose and Hb A_o (k_{-1}) (see Fig. 1.1). The rate of the Amadori rearrangement to form the ketoamine A_{Ic} (k_2) will be the third one. This step is considered to be slow and irreversible. Higgins and Bunn (32) were the first to determine these kinetic constants. The initial condensation reaction rate (all the glycosylation sites included) was first determined by in-

Table 3.4 Hematological Parameters of Red Cell Fractions from Adults and Newborn Infants

Sample	Fraction number		% Fraction	Reticulocytes (%)	MCV (fl)	MCH (pg)	MCHC (g/dl)
Adult	(Top)	1	22.6	2.3	90	29.9	31.0
		2	24.5	0.5	86	29.7	32.0
		3	28.7	0.1	85	29.0	33.0
		4	18.0	0	83	29.8	33.1
	(Bottom)	5	6.2	0	80	28.0	32.0
	Total		—	0.7	84	29.8	33.0
Cord blood	(Top)	1	27.5	4.6	119	38.2	31.0
		2	31.2	0.6	110	36.6	32.2
		3	25.7	0.4	106	36.0	32.8
		4	8.0	0.5	105	36.2	32.6
	(Bottom)	5	7.6	0	98	36.0	33.0
	Total		—	2.2	109	36.9	32.1

Source: From Elseweidy et al. (27) by permission of the C. V. Mosby Company.

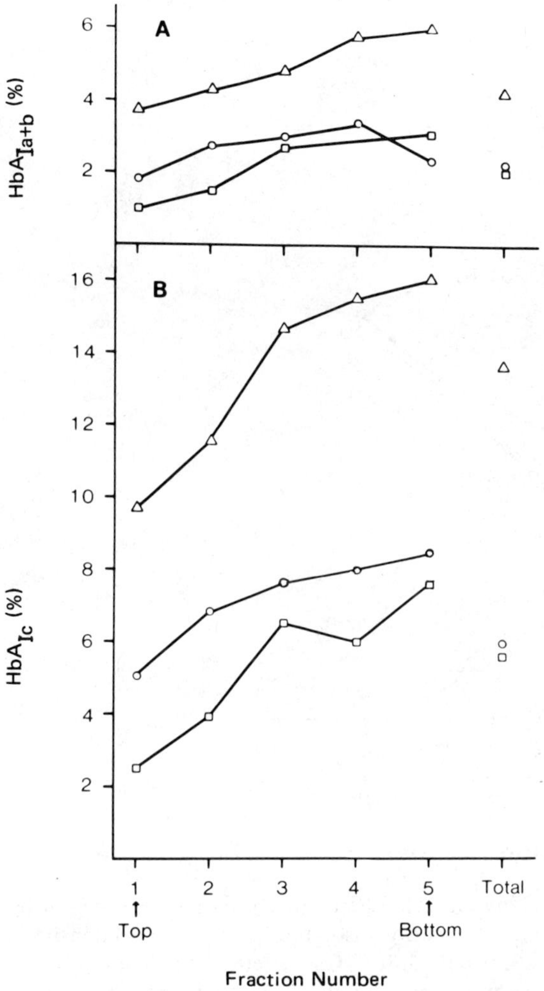

Figure 3.8 Proportions of Hb A_{Ia+b} (A) and Hb A_{Ic} (B) in red cell fractions of a normal adult (○), a White's class A diabetic patient with controlled diabetes (□), and a patient with uncontrolled IDDM (△), prepared by Dextran 40 density gradient centrifugation. From Elseweidy et al. (27) by permission of the C. V. Mosby Company.

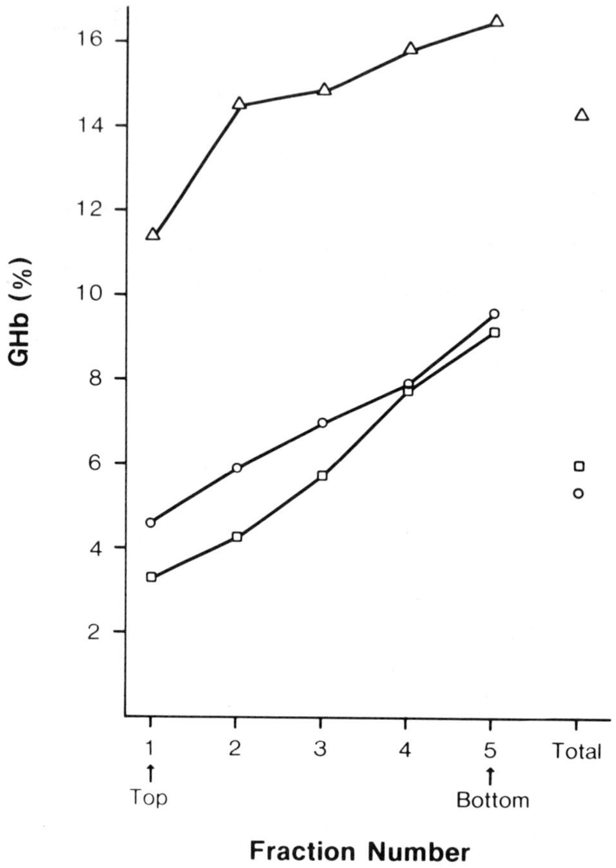

Figure 3.9 Levels of the total glycosylated hemoglobin (GHb) determined by affinity chromatography in red cell fractions isolated by Dextran 40 density gradient centrifugation from a normal adult (○), a patient with adequately controlled White's class A diabetes (□), and a patient with uncontrolled IDDM (△). Reproduced from Elseweidy et al. (27) by permission of the C. V. Mosby Company.

cubating purified D-[^{14}C] glucose (purified from commercially available product) with chromatographically purified Hb A_o (CO saturated) under physiologic conditions in the presence of cyanoborohydride, which traps the Schiff base and reduces it to a stable adduct. The rate constant ($k_1' = 0.9 \pm 0.2 \times 10^{-3}$ mM^{-1} hr^{-1}) determined in this manner represents all the sites and does not differentiate the β-chain NH_2 terminus. Partial information on the sites of glycosylation was obtained by comparing the reactivities of Hb A_o and of Hb A_{Ic}, whose β-chain NH_2-terminal groups are already blocked. To achieve this, a parallel incubation was done with Hb A_{Ic}, which revealed the contribution of all the sites except the β-chain NH_2-terminal amino groups. Then, the true rate (k_1) of glycosylation of the β-chain NH_2 terminus (formation of Hb A_{Ic}) was estimated to be 0.3×10^{-3} mM^{-1} hr^{-1}. The k_{-1} (reverse reaction) was determined from incubations carried out in the absence of cyanoborohydride. The incorporation of glucose into hemoglobin was curvilinear, lower than that in the presence of cyanoborohydride, and incorporation leveled off after 4 hr. The rate constant k_{-1} calculated from these data was 0.33 hr^{-1}. For determination of k_2, prolonged (several days) incubation of Hb A_o with D-glucose and subsequent chromatographic separation of Hb A_{Ic} was needed. Incubations were done for about 16 days with 50 mM concentration of glucose. A linear increase in Hb A_{Ic} was seen during this period. The k_2 determined in this manner was 0.0055 hr^{-1}.

Criticisms can be raised against the authenticity of using these approaches to determine the true rate constants reflecting the in vivo situations. Low Hb concentration in the incubations, using CO as the ligand, absence of 2,3-DPG in the incubations, and difficulty in determining the true k_1 are a few apparent drawbacks. Despite these reservations, the rate constants provided here could be reasonably close to those in vivo and should provide insight into the mechanisms responsible for nonenzymatic glycosylation of hemoglobins. Consideration of the various rate constants will reveal that during incubation of hemoglobin with glucose, the labile aldimine increases within a few hours to reach an equilibrium plateau. Only a minute amount of the ketoamine is formed during the initial stage, since the rate of Amadori rearrangement (k_2) is only a small fraction (about one-sixtieth) of the rate of the dissociation of the Schiff base (k_{-1}). There is a rapidly equilibrating level of the labile aldimine at any given glucose concentration. The approximate level of this labile form of the glycosylated Hb can be estimated from the rate constants. In normal red cells, about 0.5% of the total Hb is pre-A_{Ic}, that is, about 10% of the total Hb A_{Ic}. In diabetics, however, pre-A_{Ic} level should be glucose concentration dependent and should vary depending on the degree of diabetic control. Assuming an average glucose concentration of 5 mM and a red cell survival of 120 days, the rate constant could predict a Hb A_{Ic} value of 3.7% as compared to a measured value of 4%.

A different, but a more direct, approach was applied by Mortensen and Christophersen (33) to calculate k_1 and k_{-1} for the formation and dissociation of pre-A_{Ic}. They, in fact, separated the pre-A_{Ic} by isoelectric focusing, and this approach was used to monitor the formation of pre-A_{Ic} and to isolate the pre-A_{Ic} to study its dissociation. The rate constants k_1 (0.096×10^{-3} liter/mol sec^{-1}) and k_{-1} (0.10×10^{-3} liter/mol sec^{-1}) calculated in this manner were different from those reported by Higgins and Bunn (32). Despite this difference, the equilibrium constant K ($k_1/k_{-1} = K = 0.96$ liter/mol at 37°C) was nearly the same in both studies. The apparent Arrhenius activation energies for the k_1 and k_{-1} reactions are 42.5 and 46.5 kJ/degree, respecrively. Consequently, the K is predicted to be nearly temperature independent. The values of the apparent Arrhenius activation energies allow the values of the rate constants to be calculated at any temperature within the experimental temperature range. This information is of importance for a closer understanding of the mechanisms of glycohemoglobin accumulation in red blood cells.

The rate constants derived in these studies are in full quantitative agreement with in vivo studies (24) and establish that, in contrast to pre-A_{Ic}, Hb A_{Ic} is formed slowly and nearly irreversible in an almost linear fashion. McDonald and Davis (34) reported a computer simulation of a model that is independent of exact kinetic constants. This model seems to have far-reaching clinical implications. Accordingly, the maximal half-time for approach to a new equilibrium, if a patient with persistent hyperglycemia is brought to perfect control, is 8.5 weeks. Any reversibility of the glycosylation reaction or decreased red cell survival will shorten this time. A short-term loss of glycemic control causes an apparent increase in Hb A_{Ic} level. Such an increase is usually more rapid than the fall that occurs when hyperglycemia is suddenly controlled. However, short-term rises may not be measurable by Hb A_{Ic} because sustained high levels of glucose are required to affect significant increases in this component.

D. Other Factors

The nonenzymatic nature of glycosylation is evident from the simple fact that it is a slow process either in cell or in cell-free systems. Moreover, there is no significant difference in the rates of glycosylation when chromatographically purified hemoglobin, red cell hemolysate, or intact red cell is used for in vitro glycosylation studies. Although enzymes and cofactors are not known to be involved in the attachment of glucose or its intermediates to Hb, other factors, such as temperature, pH, and glucose concentration, can influence the rate of nonenzymatic glycosylation. According to Spicer et al. (35), Hb A_{Ic} increases with time, glucose concentration, and temperature. Between pH 6.5 and 9.5, no significant difference in Hb A_{Ic} synthesis was observed. However, at pH 5.0, Hb A_{Ic} formation was significantly reduced. This contradicts to some extent with the observation that the rate constant k_1' increased with increasing pH between pH 5 and 8.0 (32). However, this study does not differerentiate between the pH dependence of the β-chain NH_2-terminus glycosylation from the glycosylation of the other sites. Glucose concentration dependence of Hb A_{Ic} formation is a well-documented fact even in in vivo systems. This is reflected in the fact that Hb A_{Ic} levels correlate with the time-averaged plasma glucose concentration. The clinical utility of the Hb A_{Ic} assay emerged from this simple fact. Moreover, galactose and mannose, but not fructose, will serve as precursors to Hb A_{Ic} (35). A good substrate for hexokinase, namely, 2-deoxyglucose, and a poor substrate for this enzyme, namely, 3-O-methylglucose, are better substrates for Hb A_{Ic} than glucose, suggesting that enzymatic phosphorylation of glucose is not required for Hb A_{Ic} synthesis. It has been postulated by some investigators (13) that G6P reacts with Hb A_o first, which is then dephosphorylated to yield Hb A_{Ic}. This conclusion was made from their failure to react glucose or mannose with Hb A_o, whereas G6P was readily reacted. Therefore, it was concluded that phosphate appears necessary to orient the carbohydrate in the 2,3-DPG pocket of the Hb molecule to facilitate addition. However, evidence for this hypothesis is weakened by subsequent in vitro studies done in several laboratories showing efficient synthesis of Hb A_{Ic} from Hb A_o and glucose. However, this does not underscore the fact that sugar phosphates form adducts with hemoglobin more rapidly than glucose. In addition to G6P and FDP, Hb reacts readily with fructose 6-phosphate, ribose 5-phosphate, ribulose 5-phosphate, and glucoronic acid, but not with glucose 1-phosphate or glucose 1,6-diphosphate (13,36). Thus, the availability of an aldehyde or a ketone group is an absolute requirement for glycosylation to take place. Moreover, the rapid formation of the adduct requires the presence of an aldehyde or a ketone group separated from a negatively charged group, such as PO_4^{2-} or COO^-. Kinetics of the formation of Hb A_{Ic} analogues will be greatly influenced by the type of the sugar that is used for glycosylation purpose. The extent to which the sugars exist in the open vs. ring (hemiacetal) structure may be important to the rate of adduct formation between the sugar and hemoglobin. Of the sugars, ribose, galactose, mannose, and glucose, in decreasing order, have the highest percentage of the open structure; ribose yields the highest rate of hemoglobin glycosylation (37).

IV. GLYCOSYLATED COMPONENTS OF HUMAN FETAL HEMOGLOBIN

A. Chromatographic Analyses

Allen et al. (38) were the first to isolate the minor hemoglobin F_I from umbilical cord blood samples by Amberlite IRC-50 cation exchange chromatography. Subsequent structural analysis by Schroeder et al. (39) have indicated that Hb F_I contains two α chains and two γ chains, one of the γ chains being acetylated at the amino terminus. Stegink and his colleagues (40) have found 1.6 *N*-acetyl groups per mol of Hb F_I. Thus, no one was able to show that both the γ chains are acetylated in Hb F_I. It is possible that the Hb F_I preparations were impure, or that another chemically modified Hb, such as a glycosylated Hb, with similar chromatographic property cochromatographed with the acetylated form of Hb F_I. We, in 1979, while working with Bio-Rex 70 chromatographic separation of the Hbs in newborn infants, demonstrated that Hb F_I is heterogeneous and that it contains mostly acetylated and some glycosylated hemoglobin components as well (19).

The original Amberlite IRC-50 chromatographic procedure of Schroeder and co-workers (1,2) was modified by substituting IRC-50 resin with Bio-Rex 70 resin (Bio-Rad, Inc.) and by introducing a starting buffer (Developer 3-a) with half the molarity (0.019 M phosphate) of the original Developer 6 (19). By doing so, Hb F_I (Hb F_{Ic}, the original nomenclature "F_I" was subsequently changed to "F_{Iac}" first and then to "F_{Ic}") and pre-F_I (Hb F_{Ia+b}) zones have been separated at room temperature (Fig. 3.10). Thus, lowering the molarity of the starting buffer enabled the separation of the minor fetal hemoglobin components from the minor adult and the major adult and fetal Hbs. Since Hb F_{Ic} and Hb F_{Ia+b} zones were not present in the chromatogram of a normal adult, but were present in an HPFH homozygote, these components are, indeed, minor components of fetal Hb. Preliminary characterization indicated that Hb F_{Ia+b} zone is formed by glycosylation of Hb F_o with phosphorylated intermediates, and Hb F_{Ic} may contain, in addition to acetylated Hb F, a glucosylated (glucose adduct) component as well.

The Bio-Rex 70 chromatographic procedure was further modified by applying a linear gradient of potassium phosphate, rather than sodium phos-

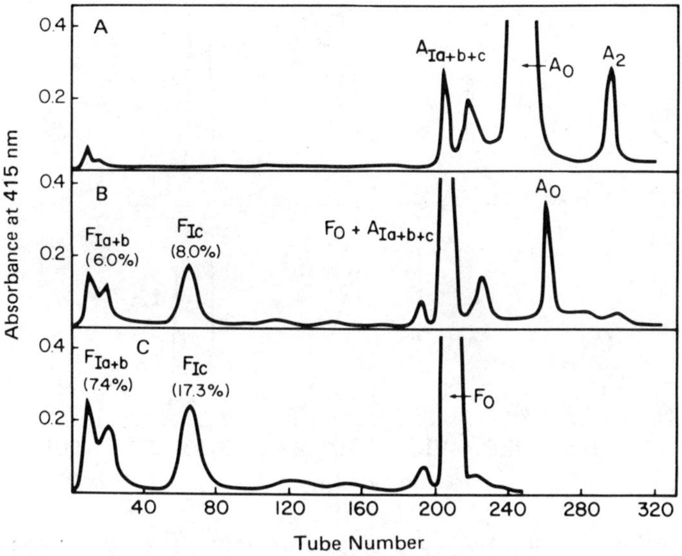

Figure 3.10 Bio-Rex 70 chromatographic separations of the hemoglobins present in freshly prepared red cell lysates of a normal adult (A), a newborn infant (B), and an adult homozygous for hereditary persistence of fetal hemoglobin (HPFH) (C). Thirty milligrams was applied to a 1 X 25 cm column and developed at room temperature with Developer 3-a as the starting buffer. A sodium phosphate gradient was developed with Developers 6, 8, and 9 (see Chap. 4). Four milliliter fractions were collected with a flow rate of 12 ml/hr. From Abraham et al. (19) with minor modifications; by permission of the Elsevier Biomedical Press.

phate, at 4°C in order to separate the minor fetal hemoglobin components to levels at which they can be characterized (21). Separated from red cell hemolysates of newborn infants and an HPFH homozygote have been Hb F_{Ia1}, Hb F_{Ia2}, Hb F_{Ib}, and Hb F_{Ic}(Fig. 3.11). The minor fetal hemoglobins in newborn infants were also separated by a high-pressure liquid chromatographic procedure (6). A Synchropak CM 300 cation exchange column was developed with Bis-Tris buffers and a sodium acetate gradient. In about 2 hr with 300 μg Hb, separation of all the minor Hbs, including a trace amount of Hb Bart's, was achieved (Fig. 3.12).

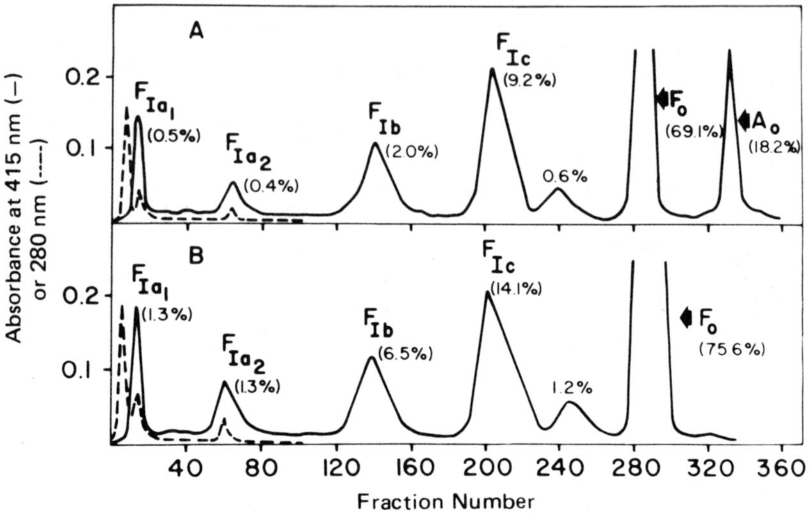

Figure 3.11 Bio-Rex 70 chromatographic separation of hemoglobins present in an umbilical cord blood sample (A) and in a blood sample from an HPFH homozygote (B). Thirty milligrams were applied to a 1 X 25 cm column and developed at 4°C using a potassium phosphate gradient at pH 6.88. The fraction size was 5 ml and the flow rate was 15 ml/hr. From Abraham (21) by permission of the Elsevier Biomedical Press.

B. Characterization of the Minor Fetal Hemoglobin Components

The Hb components isolated by Bio-Rex 70 chromatography were analyzed for Hb-bound ketoamine and phosphate (21) (Table 3.5). All the minor Hbs showed absorbance spectra typical for the complex that 5-HMF forms with TBA, with an λ_{max} at 443 nm. On the basis of this assay, the ketoamine content of Hb F_{Ia1}, Hb F_{Ia2}, Hb F_{Ib}, and Hb F_{Ic} were significantly larger than that of Hb F_o fraction. However, as expected, Hb A_{Ic}, which was used as a control, gave the highest level of the TBA reaction. Hemoglobin F_{Ic} was one of the lowest ketoamine-containing fractions, most probably due to the fact that it contains mostly acetylated γ chains. Results of phosphate analysis (Table 3.5) showed that Hb F_{Ia1}, as in Hb A_{Ia1}, contains about 4 mols of phosphorus per mol of Hb tetramer, whereas Hb F_{Ia2}, just like Hb A_{Ia2}, have 2 mol of phosphorus per tetramer. Thus, it seems that Hb F_{Ia1} and Hb F_{Ia2} are

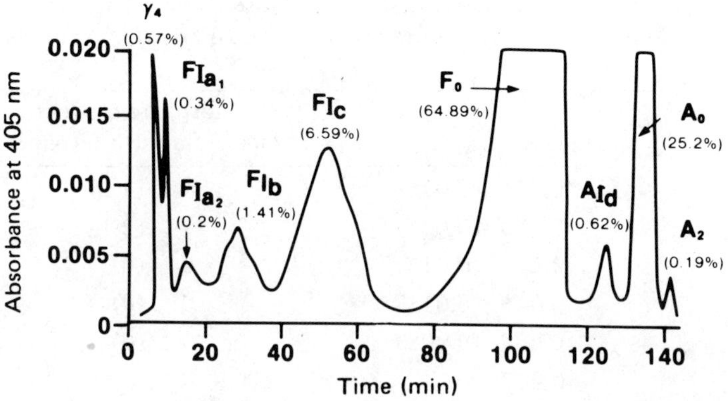

Figure 3.12 Separation of the minor hemoglobins in a newborn baby by cation exchange high-pressure liquid chromatography. Three hundred micrograms of Hb were applied to a Synchropak CM 300 column and developed at a flow rate of 1 ml/min with Bis-Tris developers and a sodium acetate gradient (see Chap. 4 for further details).

adducts of FDP and G6P, respectively, with the γ-chain NH_2-terminal amino groups. Hemoglobin F_{Ib} is a glycosylated Hb, but contains no phosphorus. Labeling of Hb F_o with [^{14}C] FDP, [^{14}C] G6P, and [^{14}C] glucose produced labeled Hb F_{Ia1}, Hb F_{Ia2}, and Hb F_{Ic}, respectively (Fig. 3.13). These studies were helpful in establishing the identities of the minor Hbs. These experiments also showed that, in addition to the radioactivity peaks under the minor Hb zones, radioactivity peaks were associated with the major Hb F_o zone. This "nonspecific binding" was only minimal with FDP and G6P. It appears that Hb F_{Ic} may be formed by both glycosylation and acetylation of γ chains. However, it should be emphasized that although glycosylated Hb F cochromatographs with Hb F_{Ic}, only a small portion of Hb F_{Ic} is normally present in the glycosylated form. Utilizing both affinity and ion exchange chromatographic methods, it has been shown that only about 5-10% of Hb F_{Ic} is in the glycosylated form (41). Moreover, it seems that the major portion of the glycosylated Hb in newborn infants is formed in vivo by glycosylation of the ε-NH_2 groups of lysyl amino acids. About 60% of the total glycosylated Hb in newborn infants is apparently formed in this manner. Recently conducted experiments (J. Jolly and E. C. Abraham, unpublished) have shown that chromatographically purified Hb F_{Ic} seems to contain a constant proportion of

Table 3.5 Results of the Colorimetric Assay for Hexoses (Using Thiobarbituric Acid) and Phosphate Analysis of Minor and Major Fetal Hemoglobin Components[a]

Hb component	Hexoses (A_{443}/mg Hb)	Phosphate content (mol P/mol Hb tetramer)
Hb F_{Ia1}	0.038 (0.035)	4.1 (4.2)
Hb F_{Ia2}	0.020 (0.025)	1.9 (2.1)
Hb F_{Ib}	0.016 (0.017)	0 (0)
Hb F_{Ic}	0.016 (0.018)	0 (0)
Hb F_o	0.009 (0.008)	0.1 (0)
Hb A_o	0.007	0.1
Hb A_{Ic}	0.094	0

[a]Hemoglobin components were isolated by Bio-Rex 70 chromatography from cord blood red cell lysates. Values between parentheses are those of the Hb fractions from the red cell lysate of an homozygote for hereditary persistence of fetal Hb.
Source: From Abraham (21) by permission of Elsevier Biomedical Press.

unmodified γ chains. The reason for this apparent hybrid structure of Hb F_{Ic} is unknown.

Functionally, the minor fetal hemoglobin components were not too different from the respective adult minor Hb components (21). Figure 3.14 gives the Hill plot of the oxygen dissociation curves for various minor fetal hemoglobin components in the presence and absence of 2,3-DPG. In the absence of 2,3-DPG, the oxygen affinities of Hb F_o, Hb A_o, Hb F_{Ic}, and Hb F_{Ib} were high and essentially the same. On the contrary, Hb F_{Ia1} and Hb F_{Ia2} had significantly lower oxygen affinity, thus strongly resembling Hb A_{Ia1} and Hb A_{Ia2}. The presence of 2,3-DPG did not influence the oxygen affinities of the four minor Hbs and of Hb F_o to any great extent; while, as expected, the P_{50} value of Hb A_o was increased. It is noteworthy that the covalent modifications with FDP and G6P raise the P_{50} or lower the oxygen affinity, although 2,3-DPG fails to show any effect due to lack of binding sites for this organic phosphate. The presence of the sugar phosphates at the central cavity of Hb F molecule shifted th conformation equilibrium to the tense or the deoxy form. It is also interesting to note that the absence of one organic phosphate binding site on the γ chains (γ143 is serine instead of histidine) did not prevent the covalent adduct formation with the sugar phosphates.

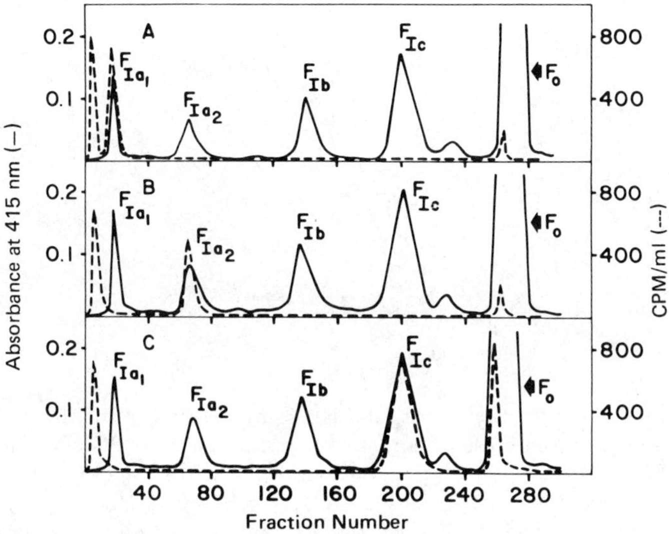

Figure 3.13 Elution profiles of in vitro formed and naturally occurring minor hemoglobin components present in the red cell lysate of an HPFH homozygote after incubation for 5 days at 4°C with (A) D-[^{14}C]fructose 1,6-diphosphate, (B) D-[^{14}C]glucose 6-phosphate, and (C) with D-[^{14}C]glucose. After gel filtration, the incubation mixture was applied on a 1 X 25 cm column of Bio-Rex 70 and developed with the same system as described in Fig. 3.11. The absorbances at 415 nm and the radioactivity of the effluent fractions were determined. From Abraham (21) by permission of the Elsevier Biomedical Press.

C. Quantitative Aspects

Minor components Hb F_{Ia+b} and Hb F_{Ic} were determined in newborn babies of nondiabetic and diabetic women, newborn infants born at term and pretern, and adults with elevated levels of Hb F due to various hematological disorders (19,27, 41-43). In adults with homozygosity for $\delta\beta$-thalassemia, β°-thalassemia, and HPFH condition and having 97-100% Hb F in their red cells, Hb F_{Ic} varied from 15.8 to 17.9% and Hb F_{Ia+b} from 7.4 to 10.1% (Table 3.6). The levels of these minor Hbs (as percentages of total Hb F) were considerably lower in adults with homozygous β^{+}-thalassemia, $\delta\beta/\beta$-thalassemia, a child with chromosomal abnormality, and normal newborn infants. Newborns of normal women had 6.3 and 10.9% (of total Hb F) of Hb F_{Ia+b} and Hb F_{Ic}, respectively. The levels of these minor components were

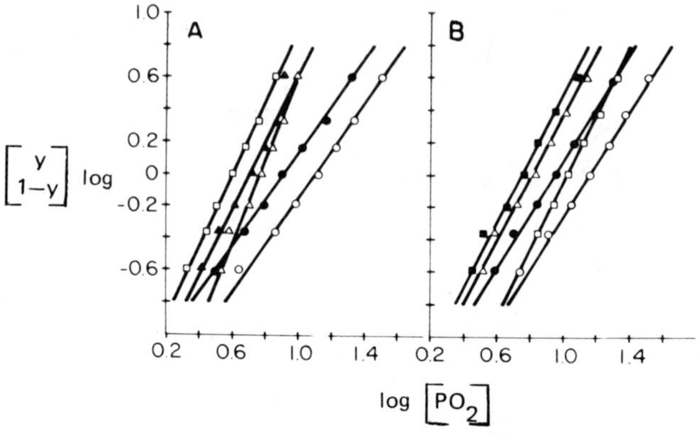

Figure 3.14 The Hill plots for the minor fetal Hb components and for the major components F_o and A_o in the presence and absence of 2 mM 2,3-DPG. (A) In the absence of 2,3-DPG: Hb F_{Ia1} (○); Hb F_{Ia2} (●); Hb F_{Ic} (△); Hb F_{Ib} (▲); both Hb F_o and Hb A_o (□). (B) in the presence of 2,3-DPG: Hb F_{Ia1} (○); Hb F_{Ia2} (●); both Hb F_{Ib} and Hb F_{Ic} (△); Hb A_o (□); Hb F_o (■). The oxygen equilibria were measured in 0.1 M Bis-Tris/Hcl, pH 7.0 at 37°C in a Hem-O-scan at a Hb concentration of 1 mM. From Abraham (21) by permission of the Elsevier Biomedical Press.

increased in newborns of mothers with IDDM (42). These minor components were also increased in term fetuses compared to those born preterm (41,43). It should be pointed out that the percentages of Hb F_{Ia+b} and Hb F_{Ic} in the newborns were significantly higher than the percentages of Hb A_{Ia+b} and Hb A_{Ic} generally found in normal adults. The difference in the levels of Hb F_{Ic} and Hb A_{Ic} is easily explainable based on the fact that Hb F_{Ic} is mainly an acetylated component. It is not clear, however, why Hb F_{Ia+b} values were so high. It is possible that some unidentified nonglycosylated components coelutes with this fraction.

V. GLYCOSYLATED COMPONENTS OF HEMOGLOBIN A_2

In addition to the major Hb A_o and a trace amount of Hb F, red cells from normal adults contain about 2.5% of Hb A_2, whereas the quantity of this Hb could be markedly increased in persons with β-thalassemia. One can expect a portion of this Hb to be present in the glycosylated form. However, the separation of the glycosylated components of Hb A_2 in red cell hemolysates is not normally feasible unless the total Hb A_2 is first purified and then the glycosylated components

Table 3.6 Percentages of Minor Fetal Hemoglobin Components in Some Hematological Disorders

Name	Genotype	Hb phenotype	Hb F_o (%)	Hb F_{Ia+b} (%)	Hb F_{Ic} (%)	Hb F_{Ia+b}/Hb F[a] (%)	Hb F_{Ic}/Hb F[a] (%)
M	Homozygous $\delta\beta$-thalassemia	FF	70.0	10.0	17.9	0.143	0.256
L	Homozygous $\delta\beta$-thalassemia	FF	72.9	9.5	15.8	0.130	0.217
J.S.	Homozygous HPFH	FF	70.6	7.4	17.3	0.105	0.245
R.H.	Homozygous β°-thalassemia	F + A_2	72.6	8.0	15.3	0.110	0.211
F.S.	Homozygous β^+-thalassemia	FA	50.7	1.8	5.3	0.036	0.105
L.J.	$\delta\beta/\beta$-Thalassemia	FA	69.2	4.8	8.6	0.069	0.124
A.D.	Trisomy D-13	FAS	42.4	1.7	4.9	0.040	0.116
B.R.	Newborn (CC)	FC	60.0	4.2	7.4	0.070	0.123
G.W.	Newborn (AA)	FA	72.3	4.1	7.3	0.057	0.101

[a]Hemoglobin F_{Ia+b} and Hb F_{Ic} were originally termed pre-F_I and F_I, respectively.
Source: From Abraham et al. (19) by permission of the Elsevier Biomedical Press.

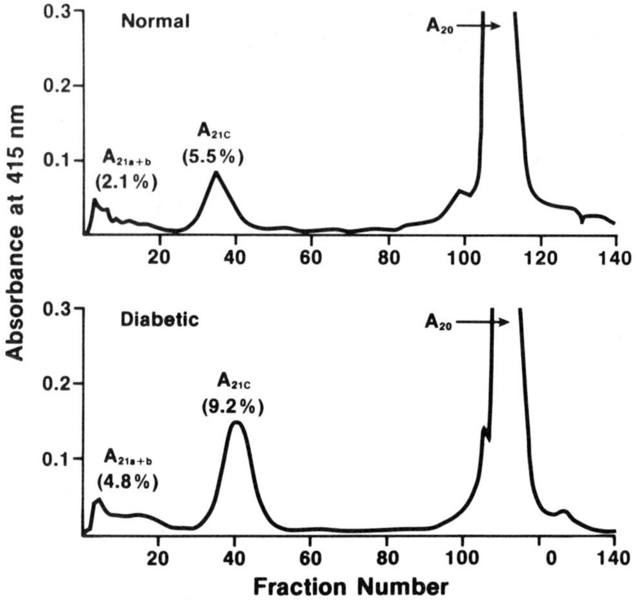

Figure 3.15 Separation of the glycosylated components of hemoglobin A_2 by Bio-Rex 70 chromatography in a normal adult and in a diabetic patient. About 25 mg of Hb A_2 was first isolated by DE-52 chromatography and then applied to a 1 X 25 cm column of Bio-Rex 70 and developed at room temperature by applying a sodium phosphate gradient with Developers 6, 8, and 10 and 5.6 ml fractions were collected.

separated. Tegos and Beulter (44) purified Hb A_2 by DE-52 chromatography and then subjected the isolated Hb A_2 to isoelectric focusing; Hb A_{2Ia}, Hb A_{2Ib}, and Hb A_{2Ic} have been separated in this manner. The quantities of all these components appeared to be significantly increased in diabetic patients. The partial identity of the minor Hb fractions was established by in vitro labeling with [^{14}C] glucose.

Glycosylated components of Hb A_2 were readily separated from DE-52 purified Hb A_2 by Bio-Rex 70 chromatography (Fig. 3.15) and cation exchange HPLC chromatography (E. Bissé and E. C. Abraham, unpublished information). To separate Hb A_{Ia+b} and Hb A_{Ic}, whole red cell hemolysates were also chromatographed under similar conditions. The mean percentages of Hb A_{2Ic} in the isolated Hb A_2 from normal adults and diabetic patients were 4.2 and 8.7%, respectively. When the Hb A_{2Ic} levels were compared with the Hb A_{Ic} levels, it became evident that Hb A_{2Ic} levels were slightly lower. Thus, it appears that Hb A_{2o} may be glycosylated to a less extent than Hb A_o.

VI. GLYCOSYLATED COMPONENTS OF HEMOGLOBIN S

A. Separation of Glycosylated Hemoglobins in Hb S Heterozygotes and Homozygotes

Around 1963, Jones and Schroeder (45), while working with Amberlite IRC-50 chromatographic separation of hemoglobins, separated a minor component termed Hb S_I from red cell hemolysate of a sickle cell anemia (SS) patient. We have attempted to separate the glycosylated hemoglobins in sickle cell heterozygotes and homozygotes by applying DEAE-Sephadex (30), CM-Sephadex (30), DEAE-cellulose (46), and Bio-Rex 70 chromatographic methods (20) and by HPLC (6). Using CM-Sephadex chromatography, Hb F_I, Hb F_o, Hb S_I, Hb A_2, and Hb S_o were separated from red cell hemolosyates of SS patients (Fig. 3.16). In this chromatographic method, 50-75 mg Hb were applied to a 0.9 × 60 cm column of CM-Sephadex and developed with Tris-maleic acid buffers of increasing pH. Hemoglobin S_I levels varied from 5.2 to 7.8%. Separation of Hb S_I was also possible by DEAE-Sephadex anion exchange chromatography. However, with both these methods, separation of Hb S_I from Hb A_o was not possible in Hb S heterozygotes. Hemoglobin A_2, Hb S_o, Hb S_I, and Hb F (eluted in that order) could be readily separated by DEAE-cellulose chromatography with glycine-KCN-NaCl developers (Fig. 3.17). The percentages of Hb S_I obtained by these methods for SS patients were rather high compared to the levels seen later with Bio-Rex 70 or HPLC methods. Menard et al. (47) and Aleyassine et al. (48) achieved the separation of Hb S_o, Hb A_o, Hb S_I, and Hb A_I in Hb S heterozygotes by agar gel electrophoresis at pH 6.3, and the proportions of the hemoglobin components were determined by scanning densitometry (see Figs. 4.26 and 4.27).

Separation of the minor Hb components A_{Ia+b}, A_{Ic}, S_{Ia+b}, and S_{Ic} in Hb S heterozygotes and F_I, S_{Ia+b}, and S_{Ic} in Hb S homozygotes was possible by Bio-Rex 70 chromatography (20) (Fig. 3.18). Glycosylated Hbs in

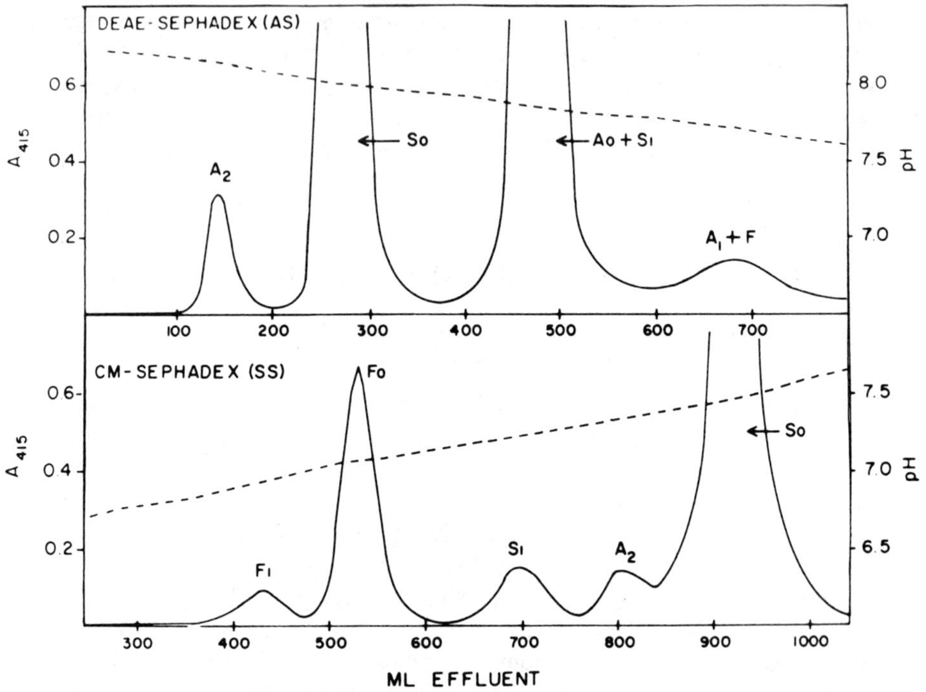

Figure 3.16 Chromatographic separation of red cell hemolysate from a SS patient on a column of CM-Sephadex,(B) and of a red cell hemolysate from a Hb S heterozygote on a column of DEAE-Sephadex (A). Fifty to 75 mg hemoglobin was applied to a 0.9 X 60 cm column of CM-Sephadex and developed with Tris-maleic acid buffers of pH varying between 6.5 and 7.8 (linearly increasing pH gradient). For DEAE-Sephadex, Tris-HCl buffers and a linearly decreasing pH gradient was used. In both the systems a flow rate of about 12 ml/hr was maintained, and 4-ml fractions were collected. Dashed lines show the pH gradient developed. From Abraham et al. (30) by permission of the Academic Press, Inc.

seven nondiabetic sickle cell anemia patients, six nondiabetic sickle cell traits (AS), four diabetic sickle cell traits, and one sickle cell anemia patient with IDDM were separated and quantitated in this manner. The percentages of Hb A_{Ia+b}, Hb A_{Ic}, Hb S_{Ia+b}, and Hb S_{Ic} were significantly increased in

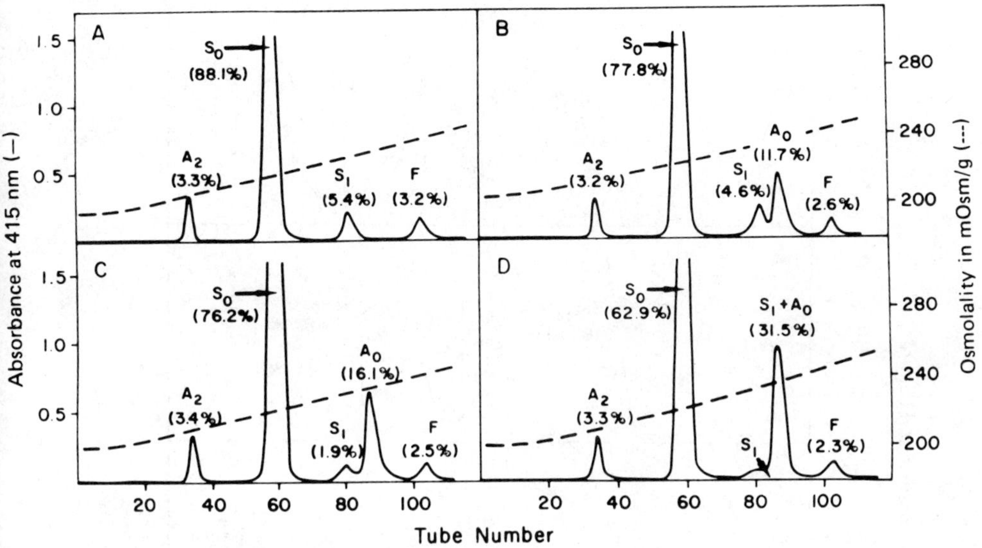

Figure 3.17 DEAE-cellulose (DE-52) chromatograms of red cell hemolysates from a sickle cell anemia patient transfused with blood from a normal donor. (A) Pretransfusion sample; (B) and (C) during transfusion; (D) after transfusion was completed. About 25 mg Hb was applied to a 1 X 25 cm column and developed with glycine-KCN-NaCl developers and a linearly increasing NaCl gradient. From Abraham et al. (46).

diabetic AS persons (Fig. 3.18 and Table 3.7). When red cell hemolysates from SS patients were chromatographed, Hb F_I (Hb F_{Ia+b+c}) was eluted in the place of Hb A_{Ia+b} and Hb F_o in the place of Hb A_{Ic}. As expected, Hb S_{Ia+b} and Hb S_{Ic} were also separated; the percentages of these minor Hbs were significantly elevated in a 20-year-old sickle cell anemia patient who also had been affected with IDDM.

For analytical purpose, the various minor Hbs could be separated by cation exchange HPLC on Synchropak CM-300 column using Bis-Tris developers and a sodium acetate gradient (6). Hemoglobin F_{Ia}, Hb F_{Ib}, Hb F_{Ic}, Hb F_o, Hb S_{Ia+b}, Hb S_{Ic}, Hb A_2, Hb S_{Id}, and Hb S_o were separated from red cell hemolysates of SS patients (Fig. 3.19). The HPLC separations were, in general, superior to Bio-Rex 70 separations. The separation of the glycosylated and acetylated fetal Hb components and Hb S_{Id} were possible only by the HPLC

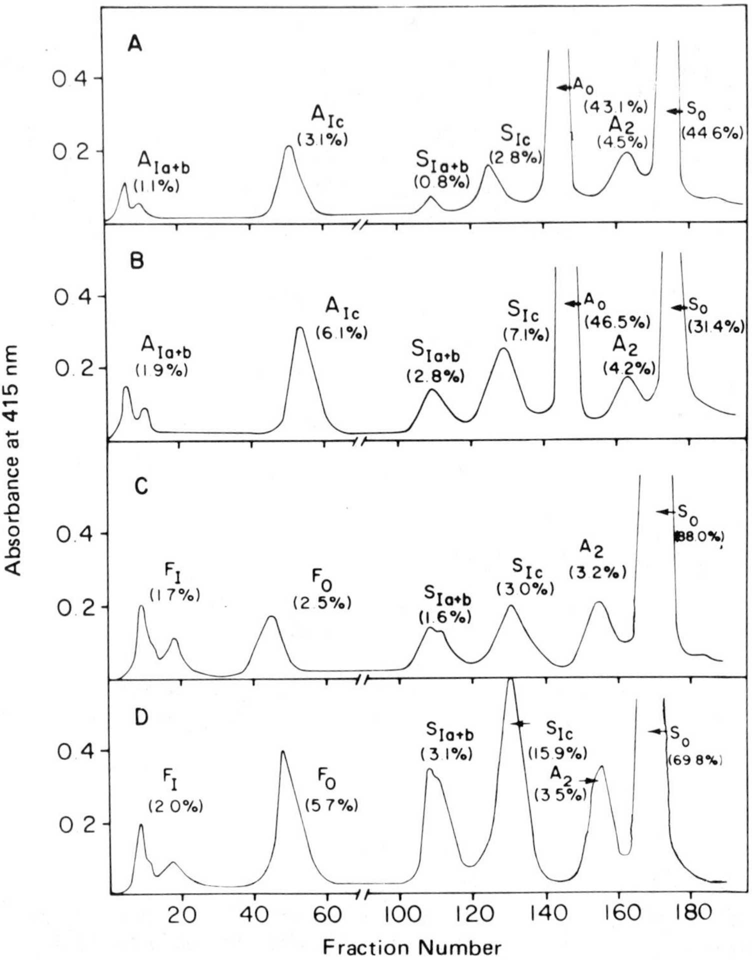

Figure 3.18 The separation by Bio-Rex 70 chromatography of the hemoglobins in freshly prepared red cell hemolysates of (A) a Hb S heterozygote (AS), (B) an AS person who has IDDM, (C) a sickle cell anemia patient (SS), and (D) a SS patient with IDDM. Thirty milligrams of Hb were applied to a 1 X 25 cm column and developed with a steadily increasing sodium phosphate gradient at room temperature. A flow rate of 8-10 ml/hr was maintained and 20-ml fractions were collected (see Chap. 4 for further details). From Abraham et al. (20) by permission of the Elsevier Biomedical Press.

Table 3.7 Composition of Hemoglobin Components of Red Cell Hemolysates from Sickle Cell Anemia Patients and Sickle Cell Traits with and without Diabetes

Patient	Condition	Hb A_{Ia+b} or Hb F_I (%)	Hb A_{Ic} or Hb F_o (%)	Hb S_{Ia+b} (%)	Hb S_{Ic} (%)	Hb A_o (%)	Hb S_o + Hb A_2 (%)
C.M.	SS-diabetic	2.0	5.7	3.1	15.9	0	73.3
C.M. (9 months later)	SS-diabetic	2.9	8.0	5.2	12.3	0	71.6
Controls (7)[a]	SS	2.2 ± 1.3[b]	6.2 ± 5.6	0.6 ± .05	2.1 ± 0.7	0	88.9 ± 7.4
D.H.	AS-diabetic	1.9	6.1	2.8	7.1	46.5	35.6
S.P.	AS-diabetic	2.1	4.0	3.9	7.5	44.9	37.6
C.C.	AS-diabetic	1.2	5.4	3.2	6.9	51.5	31.8
E.S.	AS-diabetic	2.1	7.2	2.6	7.7	48.6	31.8
Controls (6)[a]	AS	0.8 ± 0.4[b]	1.9 ± 0.9	0.7 ± 0.2	2.4 ± 0.7	50.2 ± 5.5	44.0 ± 5.4

[a]Number of persons in each control group in parentheses.
[b]Mean ± S.D.
Source: From Abraham et al. (20) by permission of the Elsevier Biomedical Press.

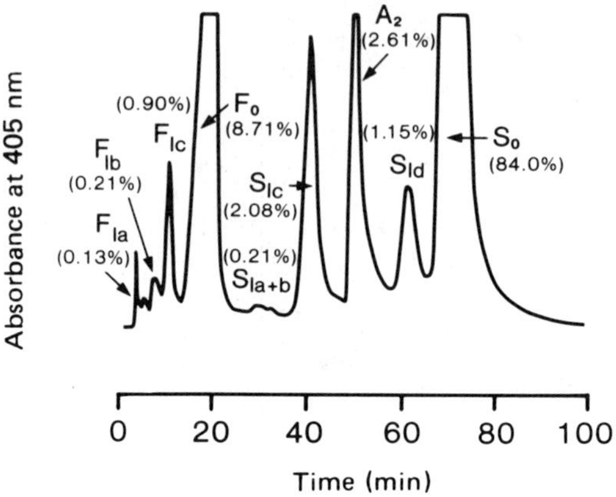

Figure 3.19 Separation by HPLC of minor hemoglobins in a SS patient. Three hundred micrograms of Hb were applied to a Synchropak CM 300 cation exchange HPLC column and developed with a gradient of sodium acetate (see Chap. 4 for further details of the gradient system).

approach. In Hb S traits, separation of Hb A_{Ia}, Hb A_{Ib}, Hb A_{Ic}, and Hb A_{Id} could be readily achieved by HPLC; however, Hb S_{Ic} cochromatographed with Hb A_o (Fig. 3.20).

B. Quantitative Aspects

The results of the Bio-Rex 70 chromatographic quantitation of the various minor Hbs in some diabetic and nondiabetic SS patients and the AS persons are summarized in Table 3.7. C.M. was a 20-year-old Black female with sickle cell anemia diagnosed at 2 years of age and with type I diabetes (IDDM) diagnosed at 11 years of age. Postprandial blood glucose values were 518 and 480 mg/dl, respectively, when the first and the second blood samples were drawn. During this period and the months previous, she showed evidence of erratic diabetic control. D.H., S.P., E.S., and C.C. were Black female teenagers with sickle cell trait who had type I diabetes diagnosed at 9-10 years of age. These persons had poorly controlled diabetic conditions at the time of blood collection. The percentages of the minor Hb components in the two samples from the diabetic SS patient were rather similar, considering that the analyses were made on materials collected 8 months apart. The levls of Hb $S_{I(s)}$ were larger than the levels of Hb $A_{I(s)}$ expressed as absolute percentages or as the per-

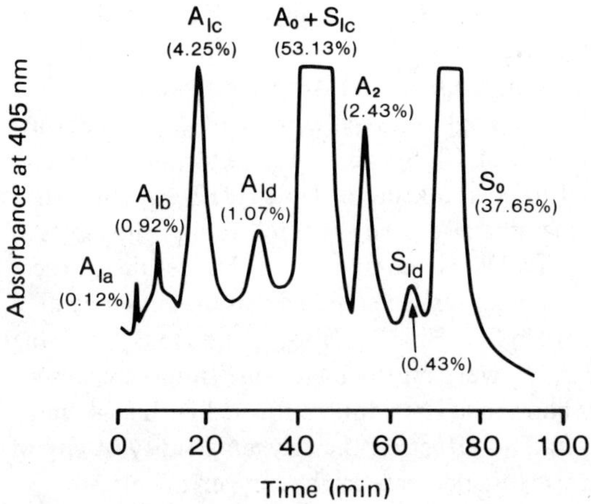

Figure 3.20 High-pressure liquid chromatographic separation of hemoglobins in a Hb S heterozygote.

centages of total Hb S or Hb A in Hb S heterozygotes. This difference was striking in the diabetic heterozygotes. Thus, it was apparent that Hb S_o was more readily glycosylated in vivo than Hb A_o. However, the sums of the percentages of Hb A_I and Hb S_I in the nondiabetic AS persons were not different from the percentage of total Hb A_I in normal adults. It should be pointed out that agar gel electrophoretic separation and quantitation of Hb $A_{I(s)}$ and Hb $S_{I(s)}$ in diabetic heterozygotes did not demonstrate any difference in the quantities of Hb $S_{I(s)}$ and Hb $A_{I(s)}$ in Hb S heterozygotes (8). The levels of Hb S_{Ic} in SS patients, either determined by Bio-Rex 70 chromatography or by HPLC (Table 3.7; see Table 4.4), were significantly lower than the Hb A_{Ic} levels in normal adults, which simply reflected the fact that the SS patients have hemolytic anemia. The mean percentages of Hb F_{Ia}, Hb F_{Ib}, and Hb F_{Ic} (calculated as the percentage of total Hb F) in the SS patients were 1.94, 3.48, and 10.44%, respectively. These levels were very similar to what is generally found in newborn infants, but lower than in HPFH homozygotes (19).

C. Identification of the Glycosylated Components

Starch gel electrophoresis at pH 9.0 showed that Hb S_{Ic} fractions from both AS and SS subjects had an electrophoretic mobility very similar to that of Hb A_o. As expected, the Hb A_{Ic} fraction migrated faster than Hb F_o and Hb A_o. The

Hb A_{Ia+b}, Hb S_{Ia+b}, Hb S_{Ia+b}, and Hb F_I fractions appeared as broad smeary bands. The levels of Hb-bound phosphate in the isolated components, Hb A_{Ia+b}, Hb S_{Ia+b}, and Hb F_I fraction, from SS and AS persons were 0.9-1.3 mol of phosphate per mol of Hb. Hemoglobin A_{Ia+b} and Hb S_{Ia+b} fractions could contain, in addition to Hb A_{Ib} or Hb S_{Ib}, both the FDP and the G6P adducts. Hemoglobin F_I seemed to be a mixture of Hb F_{Ia}, Hb F_{Ib}, and Hb F_{Ic}. Analysis for Hb-bound ketoamine also gave expected values, the largest amount being present in Hb A_{Ic} and Hb S_{Ic} components. The results of the oxygen equilibrium studies were not totally unexpected. In the presence of 2,3-DPG, the oxygen affinities of Hb S_{Ic}, Hb A_{Ic}, Hb A_o, and Hb S_o were high, but those of Hb A_{Ia+b} and Hb S_{Ia+b} were on the lower side simply because these two fractions presumably contained the adducts formed with FDP and G6P. The presence of 2,3-DPG had no effect on the oxygen affinity of any of the minor Hb fractions, in contrast to a decrease in the oxygen affinity of Hb A_o or Hb S_o.

Quantitative data have indicated that Hb S_o may be glycosylated more readily than Hb A_o. To confirm this possibility, in vitro glycosylation studies of chromatographically purified Hb F_o, Hb A_o, and Hb S_o were conducted (20). In addition, in vitro glycosylation of Hb S_o with labeled precursors aided in the identification of the glycosylated components as well. One hundred milligrams of carbon monoxide-saturated Hb in 0.1 M potassium phosphate, pH 7.0, were incubated with 20 μCi of purified [^{14}C]glucose, [^{14}C]-FDP, or [^{14}C]G6P (5 mM sugar). To determine the glucose concentration dependence of glycosylation, incubations were done with 5 to 400 mM glucose. At the end of the incubation, the reaction mixture was treated with 20 mM cyanoborohydride and subjected to Sephadex G-25 gel filtration. Each of the sugars (glucose, G6P, and FDP) was incorporated at about the same rate and extent by the three different types of hemoglobins, but the incorporation of G6P and FDP, as expected, was higher than that of glucose. Hb F_o, Hb S_o, and Hb A_o showed nearly identical concentration dependence of the glucose incorporation (Fig. 3.21). At 250 mM glucose concentration, about 1 mol of glucose was incorporated per mol of Hb after 24 hr of incubation. Thus, the results of in vitro glycosylation studies did not confirm the conclusions based on quantitative analyses that Hb S may be preferentially glycosylated in vivo. Moreover, Hb S components, which resulted from the incubation of Hb S_o with [^{14}C]FDP or [^{14}C]G6P, cochromatographed with the naturally occurring Hb S_{Ia+b} zone, and Hb S_o incubated with [^{14}C]glucose produced components that cochromatographed with Hb S_{Ic} (Fig. 3.22). Moreover, an additional radioactivity peak was

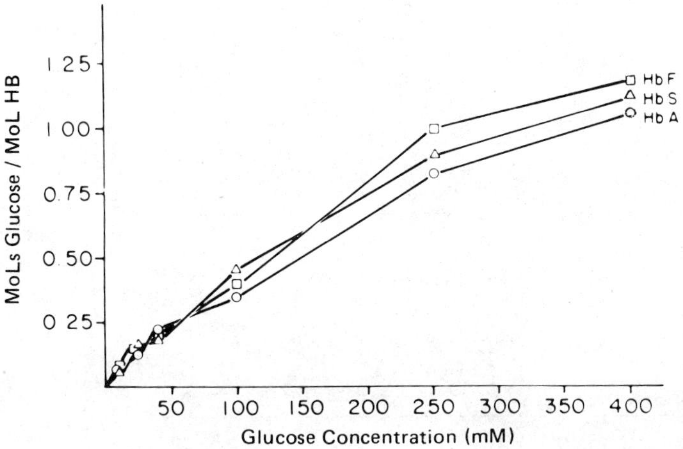

Figure 3.21 The glucose concentration dependence of glycosylation of Hb A_o, Hb F_o, and Hb S_o. From Abraham et al. (20) by permission of the Elsevier Biomedical Press.

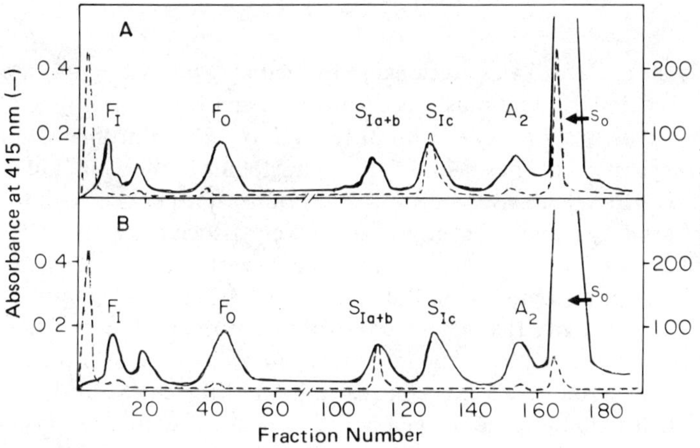

Figure 3.22 The separation by Bio-Rex 70 chromatography of the hemoglobins in a red cell hemolysate from a sickle cell anemia patient after incubation with [^{14}C] glucose (A) and with [^{14}C] glucose 6-phosphate (B). From Abraham et al. (20) by permission of the Elsevier Biomedical Press.

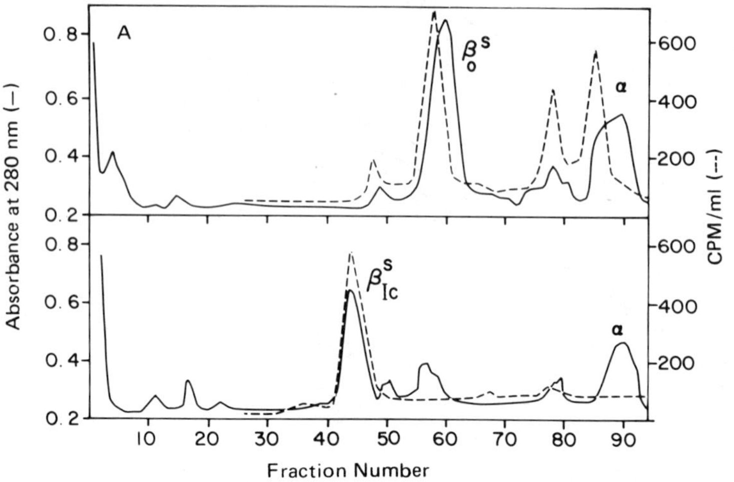

Figure 3.23 The separation by CM-cellulose chromatography of the chains of $[^{14}C]$glucose-labeled hemoglobin in the Hb S_o and Hb S_{Ic} zones. The zones were isolated by Bio-Rex 70 chromatography (see Fig. 3.22). From Abraham et al. (20) by permission of the Elsevier Biomedical Press.

associated with Hb S_o, which was presumably formed by glycosylation at sites other than the β-chain NH_2 terminus. As with Hb A_o and Hb F_o, this type of binding occurred mostly for glucose, but not for G6P or FDP. Chromatograms illustrating the separation of the chains of the hemoglobins in the $[^{14}C]$glucose-labeled Hb S_o and Hb S_{Ic} are given in Fig. 3.23. Four major peaks of radioactivity were observed. Large radioactivity zones were associated with the β chains and α chains, which, however, did not coincide with the respective absorbance peaks. These peaks were due to the binding of $[^{14}C]$glucose to lysyl residues. Other radioactivity that coincided with the absorbance peak of the pre-α zones probably resulted from the incorporation of the label into the α-chain amino-terminal groups. As expected, separation of the chains of the $[^{14}C]$glucose-labeled Hb S_{Ic} zone showed only one peak of radioactivity that matched with the absorbance peak of the β chain. An approach different from that of Bunn and his associates (17,18) was adopted to identify the sites of glycosylation. The total glycosylated hemoglobin (GHb) from red cell hemolysates was first isolated by phenylboronate-agarose affinity chromatography (49). The GHb fraction was further fractionated into Hb S_{Ic}- and Hb S_o-glycosylated components by Bio-Rex 70 chromatography. Globin was made from these Hb fractions and treated with trypsin for subsequent separation of the glycosylated tryptic peptides by phenylboronate-polyacrylamide affinity chromatography (50). The peptides purified in this manner were further separated into individual peptides by HPLC on reverse-phase columns. No significant differences between the glycosylation sites of Hb A_o and Hb S_o were noticed.

VII. GLYCOSYLATED COMPONENTS OF HEMOGLOBIN C

A. Separation of Glycosylated Hemoglobins in Hb C Heterozygotes and Homozygotes

The minor and the major Hb components present in homozygous CC patients, in SC patients, and in Hb C heterozygotes have been separated and quantitated by Bio-Rex 70 chromatography with a continuously increasing sodium phosphate gradient (51). Bio-Rex 70 methods were especially useful for isolation of the minor Hbs for subsequent analyses. Several hemoglobin components designated F_I, F_o, C_{Ia+b}, A_2, C_{Ic}, C_{Id}, and C_o were separated from blood samples of Hb C homozygotes (Fig. 3.24 and Table 3.8). The percentages of the glycosylated components Hb C_{Ia+b} and Hb C_{Ic} were, on the average, 2.4 and 4.9%, respectively. In addition, around 2.8% Hb C_{Id}, 10.5% Hb F_o, and 4.2% Hb F_I were also present in these samples. Hemoglobin A_2, which was well separated from Hb C_o gave a value of about 3.2%. In the SC patients, in addition to Hb F_I and Hb F_o, the minor components Hb S_{Ia+b} and Hb S_{Ic} have been separated; the levels of both these components were significantly elevated in the diabetic SC patient (Fig. 3.25 and Table 3.8). Hemoglobin C_{Ic}, on the other hand, was not separated from Hb S_o. It is noteworthy that the same SC patient had nearly normal levels of Hb S_{Ia+b} and Hb S_{Ic} when the analysis was repeated 1 year later after adequate control of diabetes. In Hb C heterozygotes, the separation of Hb $A_{I(s)}$ did not constitute any problem. Hb C_{Ia+b}, however, was apparently eluting with Hb A_o. Hemoglobin C_{Ic}, on the other hand, was well separated from Hb A_2, although the separation of Hb A_2 from Hb C_o was rather incomplete. The levels of Hb A_{Ia+b}, Hb A_{Ic}, Hb C_{Ic}, Hb $A_{Id1(s)}$, and Hb C_{Id} were significantly increased in the AC-diabetic person (Fig. 3.26 and Table 3.8). Separation of even the Hb A_{Id1}, Hb A_{Id2}, and Hb A_{Id3} fractions was possible with this chromatographic system. The percentages of Hb C_{Ic} were nearly the same (4.9 ± 0.4%) in all five CC patients. Interestingly, the Hb C_{Ic}

Table 3.8 Quantities of Minor Hemoglobin Components in Red Cell Hemolysates of Homozygous CC Patients, SC Patients, and Hb C Traits with or without Diabetes

Condition	Percentages (mean ± S.D.) of hemoglobin components						
	Hb F_I	Hb F_o	Hb C_{Ia+b}	Hb A_2	Hb C_{Ic}	Hb C_{Id}	Hb C_o
CC (5)[a]	4.2 ± 4.7	10.5 ± 11.5	2.4 ± 1.8	3.2 ± 0.5	4.9 ± 0.4	2.8 ± 1.0	72.0 ± 16.3
Condition	Hb F_I	Hb F_o	Hb S_{Ia+b}	Hb S_{Ic}	Hb C_{Ia+b}	Hb A_2	Hb S_o + Hb C_{Ic}
SC (17)	1.1 ± 0.5	2.4 ± 0.9	0.3 ± 0.1	1.6 ± 0.3	0.7 ± 0.2	3.5 ± 1.7	45.1 ± 2.8
SC-diabetic (1)[b] (uncontrolled)	2.2	5.1	0.7	5.4	0.9	2.3	40.4
SC-diabetic (1)[b] (controlled)	1.5	5.7	0.4	1.6	0.6	1.9	41.4

Condition	Hb C_{Id}	Hb C_o
SC (17)	2.7 ± 0.7	42.6 ± 2.0
SC-diabetic (1)[b] (uncontrolled)	3.6	38.3
SC-diabetic (1)[b] (controlled)	2.5	44.6

Condition	Hb A_{Ia+b}	Hb A_{Ic}	x	Hb A_{Id1}	Hb A_{Id2}	Hb A_{Id3}	Hb A_o + Hb C_{Ia+b}
AC (12)	1.7 ± 0.3	3.5 ± 0.5	0.5 ± 0.2	0.4 ± 0.1	1.0 ± 0.5	2.8 ± 0.01	45.9 ± 2.7
AC-diabetic (1)	2.4	8.9	0.6	1.2	2.0	3.6	37.7

Condition	Hb A_2	Hb C_{Ic}	Hb C_{Id}	Hb C_o
AC (12)	5.9 ± 0.6	2.4 ± 0.2	1.8 ± 0.9	33.2 ± 2.3
AC-diabetic (1)	6.3	4.6	3.2	29.5

[a]Number of samples analyzed in parentheses.
[b]These samples were collected from the same patient before and after adequate control of diabetes.
Source: From Abraham et al. (51) by permission of the C. V. Mosby Company.

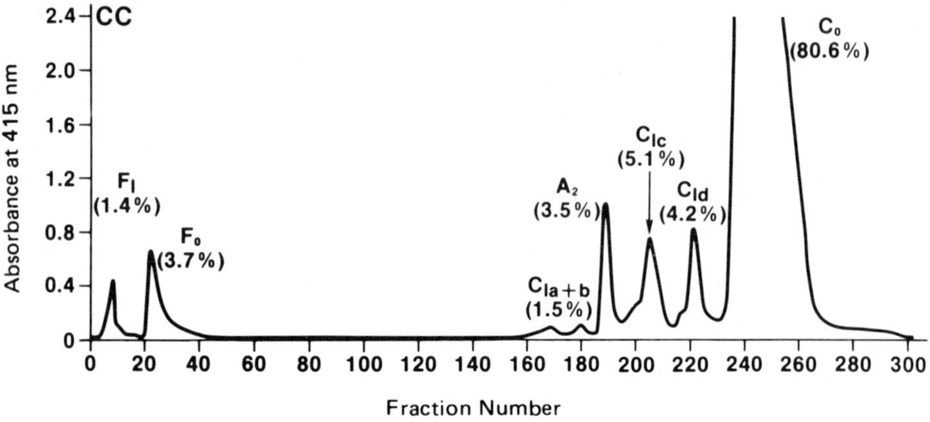

Figure 3.24 Separation by Bio-Rex 70 chromatography of the hemoglobins in red cell hemolysate from a homozygote for Hb C. Two hundred milligrams of Hb were applied to a 2 X 25 cm Bio-Rex 70 column and developed at room temperature with continuously increasing sodium phosphate gradient with Developers 6, 8, 9, and 10 (Chap. 4). A flow rate of 16-18 ml/hr was maintained and 20-min fractions were collected. From Abraham et al. (51) by permission of the C. V. Mosby Company.

values in Hb C homozygotes were significantly higher than the Hb S_{Ic} values in Hb S homozygotes (Tables 3.8 and 3.7). The percentages of Hb S_{Ic} (1.6 ± 0.3%) in nondiabetic SC patients and of both Hb C_{Ic} (2.4 ± 0.2%), and Hb A_{Ic} (3.5 ± 0.5%) in the nondiabetic Hb C heterozygotes also did not show large individual variations. Moreover, the percentages of Hb A_{Ic} (of total Hb A) and of Hb C_{Ic} (of total Hb C) were nearly the same in the AC subjects, indicating that both Hb A and Hb C may have been glycosylated at about the same rate and extent.

Separation of the glycosylated Hb components in CC and SC patients and Hb C heterozygotes was also achieved by HPLC (6). About 300 g of Hb were applied to a Synchropak CM 300 cation exchange column and developed with a linear sodium acetate gradient. The percentages of the various Hb components obtained were comparable to those determined by Bio-Rex 70 methods. Hemoglobin F_{Ia+b}, Hb F_{Ic}, Hb F_o, Hb C_{Ia+b}, Hb A_2, Hb C_{Ic}, Hb C_{Id}, and Hb C_o were separated in a CC patient (Fig. 3.27). In the SC patient, the separation of the minor fetal and sickle hemoglobins was readily possible, whereas Hb C_{Ic} was apparently not separated from Hb S_o (Fig. 3.28). In the Hb C heterozygote,

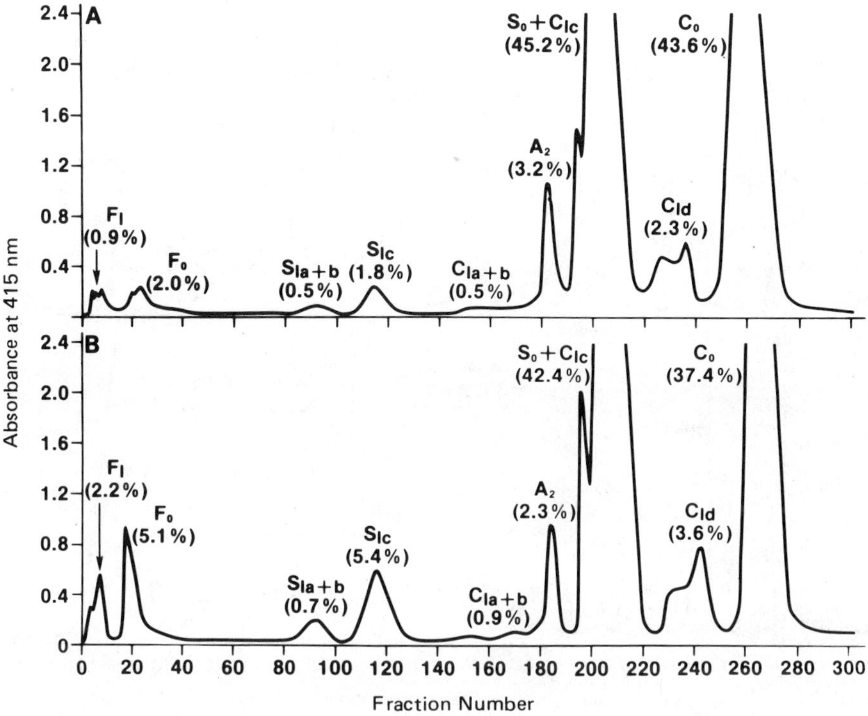

Figure 3.25 Bio-Rex 70 chromatographic separation of hemoglobins in (A) a SC patient and (B) a SC patient with IDDM before adequate control of diabetes. From Abraham et al. (51) by permission of the C. V. Mosby Company.

separation of Hb A_{Ia+b}, Hb A_{Ic}, Hb A_{Id}, Hb A_o, Hb A_2, Hb C_{Ic}, and Hb C_o were achieved (Fig. 3.29). Again, as with the Bio-Rex 70 method, the levels of Hb C_{Ic} in the CC patient (3.46%) and of Hb S_{Ic} (3.76 or 7.79% of the total Hb S) in the SC patient were higher than the Hb S_{Ic} levels in the SS patients.

Aleyassine and co-workers (48) have successfully used agar gel electrophoresis for the separation of Hb C_I and Hb A_I in four Hb C heterozygotes who had IDDM (see Figs. 4.26 and 4.28). Hemoglobin C_o, Hb C_I, Hb A_o, and Hb A_I were determined before and after a period of 3 months of therapy. Although the absolute levels of Hb A_I (5.7 to 8.5%) were higher than the levels of Hb C_I (3.9 to 6.3%), the percentages calculated per total Hb A

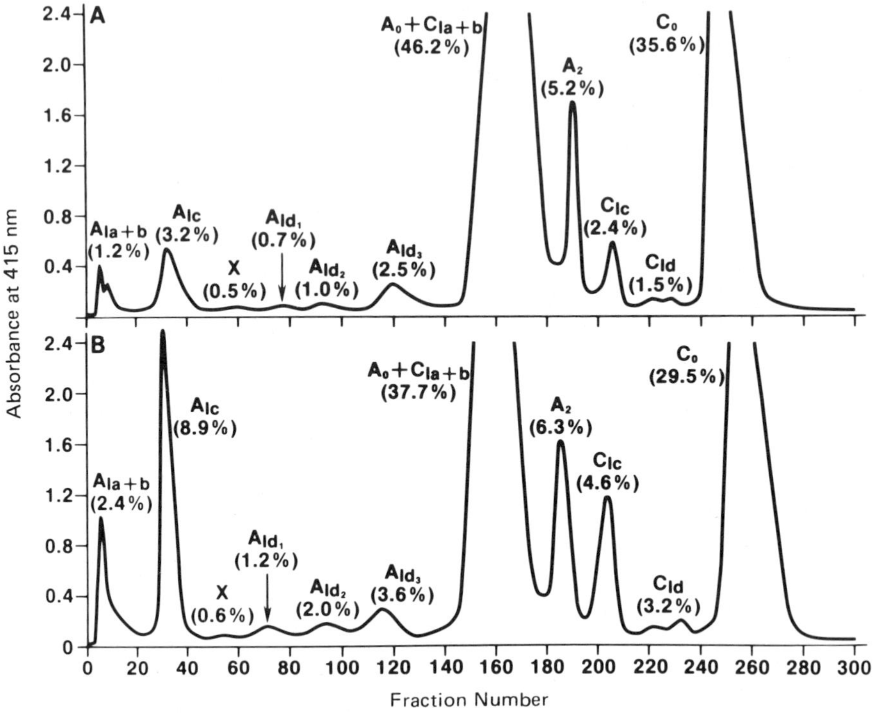

Figure 3.26 Bio-Rex 70 chromatographic separation of hemoglobins in (A) a Hb C heterozygote (AC) and (B) an AC person with IDDM before adequate control of diabetes. From Abraham et al. (51) by permission of the C. V. Mosby Company.

or Hb C were similar, again indicating that Hb A and Hb C are glycosylated at about the same rate and extent.

B. Identification of the Glycosylated Components

To identify the glycosylated Hb components separated by Bio-Rex 70 chromatography, the isolated Hb fractions were analyzed for Hb-bound ketoamine and phosphate. The Hb F_I, Hb C_{Ia+b}, and Hb C_{Ic} fractions from the CC patients contained significant amounts of ketoamine. Similarly, Hb A_{Ia+b}, Hb A_{Ic}, and Hb C_{Ic} from Hb C traits and Hb F_I, Hb S_{Ia+b}, Hb S_{Ic}, and

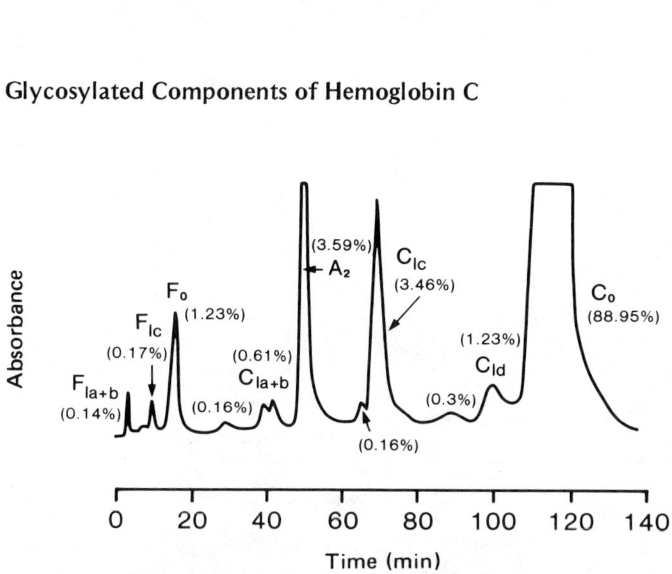

Figure 3.27 High-pressure liquid chromatographic separation of the hemoglobins in a CC patient. Three hundred micrograms of Hb were applied to a Synchropak CM 300 cation exchange HPLC column and developed with a linear sodium acetate gradient (see Chap. 4). From Abraham et al. (6) by permission of the C. V. Mosby Company.

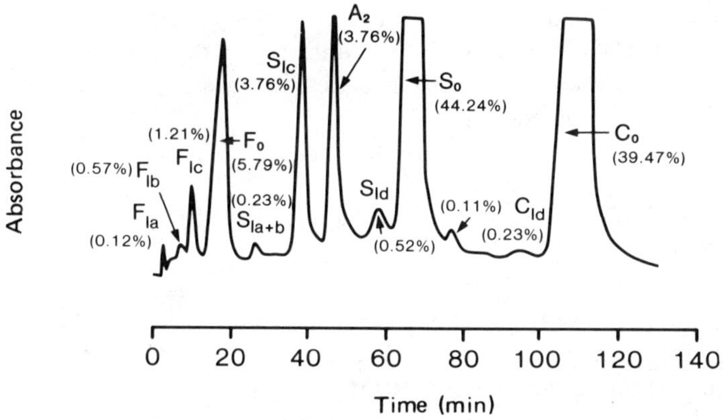

Figure 3.28 High-pressure liquid chromatographic separation of the hemoglobins in a SC patient. From Abraham et al. (6) by permission of the C. V. Mosby Company.

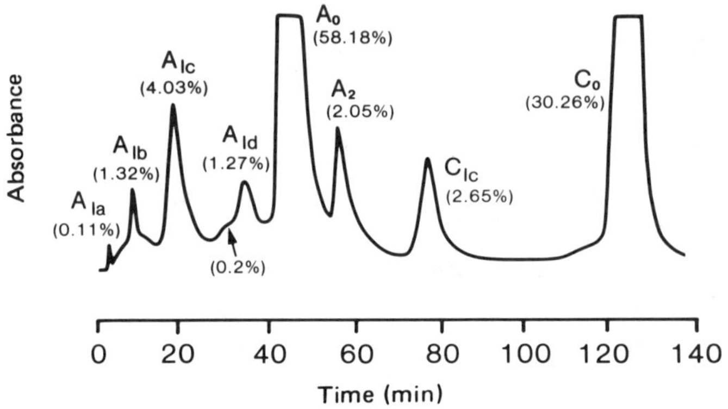

Figure 3.29 High-pressure liquid chromatographic separation of the hemoglobins in an AC person. From Abraham et al. (6) by permission of the C. V. Mosby Company.

Hb C_{Ia+b} from the SC patients also had large amounts of ketoamine. In general, Hb S_{Ic} and Hb C_{Ic} had the most detectable amounts of the sugar. In addition, Hb F_I, Hb C_{Ia+b}, Hb A_{Ia+b}, and Hb S_{Ia+b}fractions contained 2 to 4 mol of phosphorus per mol of Hb. This was indicative of the presence of FDP and G6P adducts in these Hb components. The identification process was further aided by in vitro glycosylation of Hb C_o with ^{14}C-labeled glucose, G6P, and FDP. Behavior on HPLC columns of minor Hbs purified by other chromatographic methods was relied on to identify the minor Hbs in the HPLC system. The increase in certain components in the diabetic patients also gave an indication that they were indeed glycosylated Hbs.

VIII. GLYCOSYLATED ANIMAL HEMOGLOBINS

A. Mouse

Koenig and Cerami (25) have focused their studies on adult diabetic mice (C57BL/KsJ-*db*/*db*) and the wild-type (C57BL/KsJ-+/+) mice. The minor hemoglobins were separated by Bio-Rex 70 chromatography according to the method of Trivelli et al. (16). The chromatographic separations were similar to that normally obtained for human adult red cell hemolysate. Hb A_{Ic}- and Hb A_{Ia+b}-like components were present in the diabetic and the wild-type mice; the percentages of these Hbs were increased about twofold in the diabetic (*db/db*) animals. The levels of the mouse Hb A_{Ia+b} (1.09% in the wild type and 1.73% in the diabetic) and Hb A_{Ic} (1.74 and 4.67%) were significantly lower than their human counterparts. This merely reflects a decreased red cell survival in these animals. Mice of the genotype *db/db* were normoglycemic until approximately 6 weeks of age, at which time their plasma glucose concentration rose rapidly to reach 500-600 mg/dl. Wild-type and *db/db* mice had identical Hb A_{Ic} levels for their first 10 weeks of life, after which the *db/db* mice displayed a rapid increase in the amount of Hb A_{Ic}. This rise in Hb A_{Ic} concentration was nearly parallel to, but occurred 4 weeks after, the rise in plasma glucose levels.

On the basis of NaB^3H_4 reduction of mouse hemoglobins A_o and A_{Ic}, the β chains of Hb A_{Ic} contained approximately one (0.82) borohydride-reducible linkage per monomer. The α chains of Hb A_{Ic} and both the α and β chains of Hb A_o had less than 0.04 residues per monomer. For biosynthetic studies, the *db/db* and +/+ mice were injected with $^{59}FeCl_3$. Comparison of the specific activities of Hb A_{Ic} and Hb A_o of the reticulocytes from both the *db/db* and +/+ animals revealed a lower specific activity in the mouse Hb A_{Ic} fraction than in the Hb A_o fraction. As in humans, this reflected a synthesis of Hb A_{Ic} from Hb A_o in the postreticulocyte stage. Thus, the gene *db* in the house mouse provides an experimental animal model for the human disease diabetes mellitus. This gene is an autosomal recessive mutation that, in the homozygous state, resembles diabetes mellitus in many ways, including the glycosylated Hb pattern.

B. Rhesus Monkey

One of the greatest advantages in using rhesus monkey for glycosylated hemoglobin studies is that like humans, this animal possesses a single major component of hemoglobin. Soloway et al. (52) have separated the glycosylated hemoglobins in red cell hemolysates of rhesus monkey utilizing Bio-Rex 70 resin in both high-pressure liquid chromatography (HPLC) and in macrochromatography with NaCl gradient. By HPLC, 1.8% Hb A_{Ia+b} and 3.9% Hb A_{Ic} have been separated in rhesus monkey, whereas red cell hemolysate from a normal adult under similar conditions separated 1.8% Hb A_{Ia+b} and 4.9% Hb A_{Ic}. With conventional Bio-Rex 70 chromatography, the minor Hbs Were further separated into Hb A_{Ia1}, Hb A_{Ia2}Hb A_{Ib1}, Hb A_{Ib2}, Hb A_{Ib3}, and Hb A_{Ic}.

The TBA test was the primary approach used to detect the presence of carbohydrate in the isolated peaks. The product of the TBA reaction in the rhesus monkey, Hb A_{Ic}, gave the typical absorption spectrum of the human Hb A_{Ic}. The monkey Hb A_o was apparently split into two peaks termed Hb A_{o1} and Hb A_{o2}. Hemoglobin A_{o1} contained carbohydrate but with less TBA reaction (absorbance at 443 nm) compared to Hb A_{Ic}. Hemoglobin A_{o2} fraction, on the other hand, contained no detectable ketoamine. It appears that Hb A_{o1} represents the glycosylated components that are formed by the glycosylation at the α-chain amino-terminal groups and ϵ-NH_2 groups of lysines.

The results of biosynthetic studies on these animals by injection of ^{59}Fe showed that the specific activity of rhesus Hb A_{o2} rose within 5 days of injection to its plateau value and fell slowly thereafter. The specific activity of Hb A_{o1} was slightly less than that of Hb A_{o2} until day 38. Hemoglobin A_{Ic} accumulated specific activity slowly and almost linearly for at least 51 days, equaling that of Hb A_{o2} at day 43 and exceeding it thereafter. These results are in agreement with the biosynthetic studies in humans where the specific activity of human Hb A_{Ic} equaled that of Hb A_o at day 60 (24). The specific activities of the three Hb A_{Ib} minor components of rhesus monkey increased more slowly than rhesus Hb A_{Ic}. These data suggest that rhesus Hb A_{Ib} minor components may be the result of further modification of Hb A_{Ic}; the slow nature of their accumulation is indicative of nonenzymatic process.

C. Baboon

Glycosylated minor hemoglobins in baboon (*Papio anubus*) have been separated by Alperin et al. (53) with macro- and microchromatographic methods utilizing Bio-Rex 70 cation exchange resin (21). The separations were achieved on normal baboons and on those induced to be diabetic with pancreatectomy. Baboon hemolysate contained a single major Hb component with an electrophoretic mobility between human Hb A and Hb F. Minor baboon hemoglobins A_{Ia} and A_{Ib} (A_{Ia+b}) and A_{Ic} were separated by Bio-Rex 70 macrochromatography as three early eluting components. However, when microcolumns were used, only one fast eluting Hb Component, i.e., Hb A_I, was seen. Thus, the separations were very similar to the human system. The percentages of Hb A_{Ia+b} and Hb A_{Ic} in the baboon controls were 1.53 and 2.40%, respectively, whereas in diabetic baboons, these values were increased to 2.63 and 5.86%. It is notable that the mean levels of the total Hb A_I or Hb A_{Ic} in the normal and diabetic baboons were approximately one-half the mean levels of the human counterparts. Since plasma glucose concentrations in normal baboons and humans are comparable, this difference may reflect the difference in red-cell life span between man (100-120 days) and baboon (30-60 days).

D. Rabbit

Glycosylated Minor Hb components were separated by Bio-Rex 70 chromatography and the total glycosylated Hb (GHb) by affinity chromatography in normal rabbits and in rabbits made diabetic by alloxan treatment (R. E. Perry and E. C. Abraham, unpublished). Rabbits were made diabetic by intravenous injection of alloxan at a rate of 100 mg per kg body weight. Seven days after the injection of alloxan, plasma glucose level was 590 mg/dl. Significant increase in GHb was noticed as early as 7 days after the injection, and the levels of GHb rose from 3.3 to 6.6% over 21 days and stayed around that level during the next 2 weeks. Thirty-five days after the first injection, an additional dose of alloxan was given to the test animal; within 17 days (total 52 days) after the injection, the plasma glucose had peaked off around 850 mg/dl and GHb was around 9%. Insulin treatment was initiated on day 70, which resulted in a drop in plasma glucose to around 130 mg/dl; this level was maintained over a period of 54 days, and the GHb levels gradually decreased from 9.3% to 4.0% during this period.

The various hemoglobins in the diabetic and in the nondiabetic control rabbits were also separated by Bio-Rex 70 chromatography with linearly increasing sodium phosphate gradient. Several rabbit minor hemoglobins, termed Hb A_{Ia1}, Hb A_{Ia2}, Hb A_{Ib1}, Hb A_{Ib2}, Hb A_{Ic}, and Hb A_{Id}, have been separated from the blood of normal and diabetic animals; the percentages of these hemoglobins were 0.48, 0.36, 0.5, 0.57, 3.3, and 0.8%, respectively, in the normal animal, and the percentages of these Hbs were increased about two-fold in the diabetic animal. Hemoglobin components were analyzed for protein-bound ketoamine by the colorimetric assay and for the total glycogroups by a fluorometric assay for formaldehyde released from the Hb-bound carbohydrate. Each Hb component was also analyzed for phosphate content. On the basis of the number of glyco groups and phosphate groups per $\alpha_2\beta_2$ tetramer, it was concluded that rabbit Hb A_{Ia1}, Hb A_{Ia2}, and Hb A_{Ic} are similar to their human counterparts. Based on electrophoretic and chromatographic analyses, rabbit hemolysate contained a single major Hb component. However, it was noteworthy that an additional component was present in about 10% of the total Hb and appeared just ahead of the rabbit Hb A_o. This component, which was not well separated from Hb A_o, also contained moderate amounts of ketoamine. It is not certain whether this minor Hb represents those components formed by glycosylation of sites other than the β-chain NH_2-terminal groups.

LIST OF ABBREVIATIONS

Bis-Tris	bis(2-hydroxyethyl)iminotris(hydroxymethyl)methane
CM	carboxymethyl
DEAE	diethylaminoethyl
FDP	fructose-1,6-diphosphate
G6P	glucose-6-phosphate
GHb	glycosylated hemoglobin
5-HMF	5-hydroxymethylfurfural
HPLC	high-pressure liquid chromatography
IDDM	insulin-dependent diabetes mellitus
ISC	irreversibly sickled cell
MCH	mean cell hemoglobin
MCHC	mean cell hemoglobin concentration
MCV	mean cell volume
TBA	thiobarbituric acid

REFERENCES

1. M. D. Clegg and W. A. Schroeder, *J. Am. Chem. Soc., 81:* 6065 (1959).
2. A. G. Schnek and W. A. Schroeder, *J. Am. Chem. Soc., 83:* 1472 (1961).
3. M. J. McDonald, R. Shapiro, M. Bleichman, J. Soloway, and H. F. Bunn, *J. Biol. Chem., 253:* 2327 (1978).
4. E. C. Abraham, M. Stallings, A. Abraham, and R. Clardy, *Biochim. Biophys. Acta, 744:* 335 (1983).
5. T. H. J. Huisman, J. B. Henson, and J. B. Wilson, *J. Lab. Clin. Med., 102:* 163 (1983).
6. E. C. Abraham, A. Abraham, and M. Stallings, *J. Lab. Clin. Med. 104:* 1027 (1984).
7. W. R. Holmquist and W. A. Schroeder, *Biochemistry, 5:* 2489 (1966).
8. R. M. Bookchin and P. M. Gallop, *Biochem. Biophys. Res. Commun., 32:* 86 (1968).
9. H. F. Bunn, D. N. Haney, K. H. Gabbay, and P. M. Gallop, *Biochem. Biophys. Res. Commun., 67:* 103 (1975).
10. R. J. Koenig, S. H. Blobstein, and A. Cerami, *J. Biol. Chem., 252:* 2992 (1977).
11. R. Flückiger and K. H. Winterhalter, *FEBS Lett., 71:* 356 (1976).
12. D. N. Haney and H. F. Bunn, *Proc. Natl. Acad. Sci., USA, 73:* 3534 (1976).
13. V. J. Stevens, H. Vlassara, A. Abati, and A. Cerami, *J. Biol. Chem., 252:* 2998 (1977).

14. R. Krishnamoorthy, G. Gacon, and D. Labie, *FEBS Lett., 77:* 99 (1977).
15. A. M. Dozy and T. H. J. Huisman, *J. Chromatogr., 40:* 62 (1969).
16. L. A. Trivelli, H. M. Ranney, and H. T. Lai, *N. Engl. J. Med., 284:* 353 (1971).
17. H. F. Bunn, R. Shapiro, M. McManus, L. Garrick, M. J. McDonald, P. M. Gallop, and K. H. Gabbay, *J. Biol. Chem., 254:* 3892 (1979).
18. R. Shapiro, M. J. McManus, C. Zalut, and H. F. Bunn, *J. Biol. Chem., 255:* 3120 (1980).
19. E. C. Abraham, N. D. Cope, N. N. Braziel, and T. H. J. Huisman, *Biochim. Biophys. Acta, 577:* 159 (1979).
20. E. C. Abraham, M. Stallings, B. F. Cameron, and T. H. J. Huisman, *Biochim. Biophys. Acta, 625:* 109 (1980).
21. E. C. Abraham, *Biochim. Biophys. Acta, 667:* 108 (1981).
22. H. F. Bunn and R. W. Briehl, *J. Clin. Invest., 49:* 1088 (1970).
23. A. Arnone, *Nature (London), 237:*146 (1972).
24. H. F. Bunn, D. N. Haney, S. Kamin, K. H. Gabbay, and P. M. Gallop, *J. Clin. Invest., 57:* 1652 (1976).
25. R. J. Koenig and A. Cerami, *Proc. Natl. Acad. Sci., USA, 72:* 3687 (1975).
26. S. Panzer, G. Kronik, K. Lechner, P. Bettelheim, E. Neumann, and R. Dudczak, *Blood, 59:* 1348 (1982).
27. M. M. Elseweidy, M. Stallings, and E. C. Abraham, *J. Lab. Clin. Med., 102:* 628 (1983).
28. C. A. Meyering, A. L. M. Israels, T. Sebens, and T. H. J. Huisman, *Clin. Chim. Acta, 5:* 208 (1960).
29. J. F. Fitzgibbons, R. D. Koler, and R. T. Jones, *J. Clin. Invest., 58:* 820 (1976).
30. E. C. Abraham, D. Walker, M. Gravely, and T. H. J. Huisman, *Biochem. Med., 13:* 56 (1975).
31. M. M. Elseweidy and E. C. Abraham, *Am. J. Hemat., 16:* 375 (1984).
32. P. J. Higgins and H. F. Bunn, *J. Biol. Chem., 256:* 5204 (1981).
33. H. B. Mortensen and C. Christophersen, *Biochim. Biophys. Acta, 707:* 154 (1982).
34. J. M. McDonald and J. E. Davis, *Human Pathol., 10:* 279 (1979).
35. K. M. Spicer, R. C. Allen, D. Hallett, and M. G. Buse, *J. Clin. Invest., 64:* 40 (1979).
36. H. F. Bunn, K. H. Gabbay, and P. M. Gallop, *Science, 200:* 21 (1978).
37. R. Dolhofer and O. H. Wieland, *FEBS Lett., 85:* (1978).
38. D. W. Allen, W. A. Schroeder, and J. J. Balog, *J. Am. Chem. Soc., 80:* 1628 (1958).
39. W. A. Schroeder, J. T. Cua, G. Matsuda, and W. D. Fenninger, *Biochim. Biophys. Acta, 63:* 532 (1962).
40. L. D. Stegink, P. D. Meyer, and M. D. Brummel, *J. Biol. Chem., 246:* 3001 (1971).

41. E. C. Abraham, M. Stallings, A. Abraham, and M. M. Elseweidy, *Hemoglobin, 7:* 449 (1983).
42. H. E. Fadel, A. Reynolds, M. Stallings, and E. C. Abraham, *Am. J. Obs. Gyn., 139:* 397 (1981).
43. H. E. Fadel and E. C. Abraham, *Am. J. Obs. Gyn., 141:* 704 (1981).
44. C. Tegos and E. Beutler, *Blood, 56:* 571 (1980).
45. R. T. Jones and W. A. Schroeder, *J. Chromatog., 10:* 421 (1963).
46. E. C. Abraham, A. Reese, M. Stallings, and T. H. J. Huisman, *Hemoglobin, 1:* 27 (1976-1977).
47. L. Menard, M. E. Dempsen, L. A. Blankstein, H. Aleyassine, M. Wacks, and J. S. Soeldner, *Clin. Chem., 26:* 1598 (1980).
48. H. Aleyassine, R. J. Gardiner, L. A. Blankstein, and M. E. Dempsey, *Clin. Chem., 27:* 472 (1981).
49. E. C. Abraham, R. E. Perry, and M. Stallings, *J. Lab. Clin. Med., 102:* 187 (1983).
50. M. Brownlee, H. Valssara, and A. Cerami, *Diabetes, 29:* 1044 (1980).
51. E. C. Abraham, B. F. Cameron, A. Abraham, and M. Stallings, *J. Lab. Clin. Med., 104:* 602 (1984).
52. J. Soloway, M. McDonald, H. F. Bunn, F. Aun, R. Cole, and J. S. Soeldner, *J. Lab. Clin. Med., 93:* 962 (1979).
53. J. B. Alperin, P. A. Down, and L. C. Stout, *Acta Haematol., 61:* 334 (1979).

4

Methods for Determination of Glycosylated Hemoglobins

I. COLUMN CHROMATOGRAPHY ON CATION EXCHANGER AMBERLITE IRC-50 OR BIO-REX 70

A. Introduction

Proteins contain ionizable groups with a wide range of ionization constants (Chap. 2). For this reason ion exchange chromatography has played an important role in the separation and purification of proteins. Taking advantage of the possible differences in molecular weights, proteins can also be separated by molecular sieve chromatography. However, hemoglobins are one group of proteins where such differences are rarely found. The separation on ion exchange chromatography is obtained by reversible adsorption. Ion exchange separations are done mainly in two stages. The first stage is sample application and adsorption; the unbound proteins are washed out using a column volume of starting developer (buffer). In the second stage, the bound proteins are separated from each other and eluted from the column in the order in which they are separated on the column. The separation is possible because different proteins have different affinities for the ion exchanger due to differences in their net charge. These affinities in turn can be controlled by varying conditions, such as pH and ionic strength of the developers used for equilibrating the column and for eluting the various proteins bound to the column. Enough differences in net charges are normally observed in various genetically determined normal or abnormal hemoglobins and in modified hemoglobins such as glycosylated and acetylated hemoglobins.

B. The Nature of the Resin

Ion exchangers may be described as cation exchangers and anion exchangers, and each of these in turn as weak and strong ion exchangers. Dowex-50, for instance, is a strong cation exchanger having sulfonated cross-linked polystyrene. Dowex-1, on the other hand, contains quaternary ammonium groups and is a strong anion exchanger. Weak anion exchangers may have primary or secondary amino groups, and weak cation exchangers may have carboxyl groups. In most occasions, when working with intact proteins, it may be necessary to use weak ion exchangers so that near-physiologic pH conditions can be used. Amberlite IRC-50 or Bio-Rex 70 is a cation exchanger of cross-linked acrylic resin with carboxylic groups. The partial structure of the resin matrix is shown in Fig. 4.1. The pK of carboxylic groups of this resin is 6.1. This cation exchanger is the most widely used resin for the separation of various glycosylated hemoglobin components. The original Amberlite IRC-50 (200-400 mesh in the hydrogen form, Rom & Haas Co., Philadelphia, Penn.) or a relatively pure product Bio-Rex 70 (200-400 mesh, sodium form, Bio-Rad Laboratories, Richmond, Calif.) is commonly used.

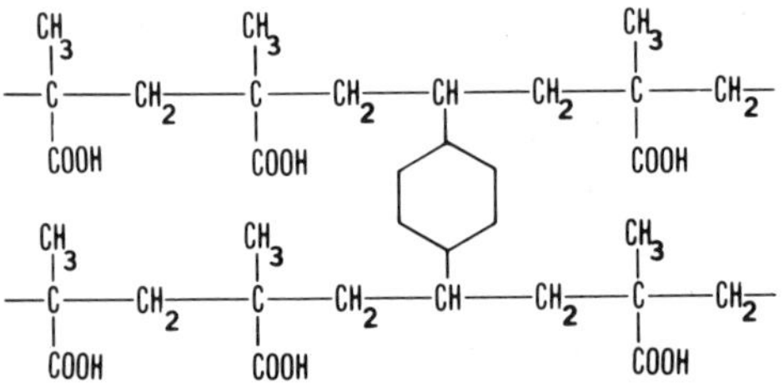

Figure 4.1 The partial structure of the resin matrix of Amberlite IRC-50 or Bio-Rex 70.

C. Preparation of the Ion Exchanger

Amberlite IRC-50 requires several steps of treatment with acid, alkali, water, and buffer before it will be ready for using as packing material for liquid column chromatography. The resin in the hydrogen form is sifted wet, and the portion that passes through a 200-mesh sieve and is retained by a 250-mesh is used. After being sifted, the resin is washed first with 3 N HCl and then with water and suspended in the appropriate buffer. The suspension is mechanically stirred, and the pH is adjusted to the original pH of the buffer with aqueous 40% sodium hydroxide at 15-min intervals; stirring is continued for several hours thereafter. The resin is washed thoroughly with the buffer and then resuspended in a sufficient volume of the buffer so that volume of the supernatant buffer is twice the volume of the settled resin. After a column has been poured with this resin, the developer is passed through at 5 to 10 ml/hr for 4 or 5 days at room temperature until the pH of the influent and the effluent are equal. The Amberlite IRC-50 is seldom used today, except by some commercial laboratories who prefer this resin to the more expensive and the prepurified Bio-Rex 70.

Bio-Rex 70, which is in the sodium form, does not require any purification or washing with acid. About 200 g of the dry material is suspended in 500 ml of Developer 9 (0.15 M sodium phosphate, pH 6.58) (Table 4.1 and Refs. 1-3), and the pH of the slurry is adjusted to the original pH of the buffer with phosphoric acid while the slurry is stirred mechanically. The slurry is left to settle for half an hour, and the supernatant is decanted. The resin is resuspended in the buffer and decanted again (pH adjusted only once). This process is repeated twice. The final product before packing the column has 1 part resin and 2 parts developer (v/v). Columns are packed with this suspension and equilibrated by passing 10 column volumes of the starting buffer (Developer 6 or Developer 3-a). It should be emphasized that irrespective of the type of sample to be chromatographed or the starting buffer used, Bio-Rex 70 resin is initially suspended in Developer 9, and the washings are done with the same buffer until the column is packed. The size of the columns will be reduced by 3 to 5 cm during initial and repeated equilibrations. Therefore, about a 30-cm column is packed first, which should give about a 25-cm column to work with. For reequilibration of the column after each use, five column volumes of a washing buffer (Developer 3-a diluted 1:1 with distilled water) are passed through it, after which it is equilibrated with a similar volume of the starting buffer.

Table 4.1 Composition of Developers Used in Bio-Rex 70 Column Chromatography[a]

Developer no.	$NaH_2PO_4 \cdot H_2O$ (g/liter)	Na_2HPO_4 (g/liter)	KCN (g/liter)	Phosphate (M)	pH[b]
3-a	2.30	0.59	0.33	0.019	6.75
6	4.59	1.18	0.65	0.038	6.73
8	9.18	2.36	0.65	0.076	6.52
9	14.35	6.52	0.65	0.150	6.58
10	28.7	13.04	0.65	0.300	6.50

[a]Developers 3-a, 6, 8, and 9 were described in Ref. 2 and Developer 10 in Ref. 3.
[b]pH values are indeed the measured values and no pH adjustment is recommended.

D. Methods of Development

Two types of development (elution) are normally followed for ion exchange chromatography. One type is "stepwise elution" in which each developer is followed by a different developer and an abrupt or "stepwise" change in conditions occur. If the changes in conditions, such as pH or ionic strength, are gradual, the method of elution is called "gradient elution." One way of achieving a gradient, e.g., in ionic strength, is by adding a solution of one concentration to a second solution of different, but lower, concentration, and the second solution is withdrawn at the rate equal to that of the addition of the first solution. The basic unit for one of the devices for gradient elution is a "constant-volume" mixer. Usually a flask having a glass stopper joint with inlet and outlet tubes and a magnetic stirrer at the bottom is used for this purpose (Figs. 4.2 and 4.3) (4). The mixer is initially filled with one solution (solution 1), and a second solution (solution 2), supplied from another container (a separatory funnel), enters the mixer at the same rate as the solution is withdrawn from the mixer. The gradient changes only slowly after a volume equal to twice the volume of the mixer has been withdrawn. This happens because the gradient is convex, with a greater initial slope that constantly decreases. By replacing solution B, after an appropriate quantity of it has been used up, with another solution (say solution 3) of higher ionic strength, the gradient can be altered significantly. In fact, there is no limit to how many different solutions can be supplied in this manner, and a linearly increasing gradient can be produced in this fashion. The nature of the gradient, i.e., small (shallow) or large (steep), will depend on the size of the mixer and the difference in the ionic strengths

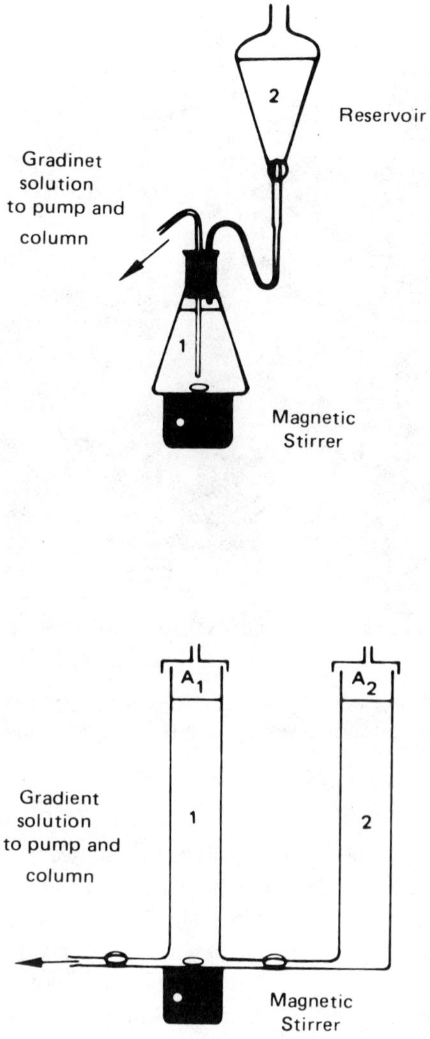

Figure 4.2 Apparatus for the development of gradients for gradient-elution chromatographic systems. Courtesy of Schroeder and Huisman (4).

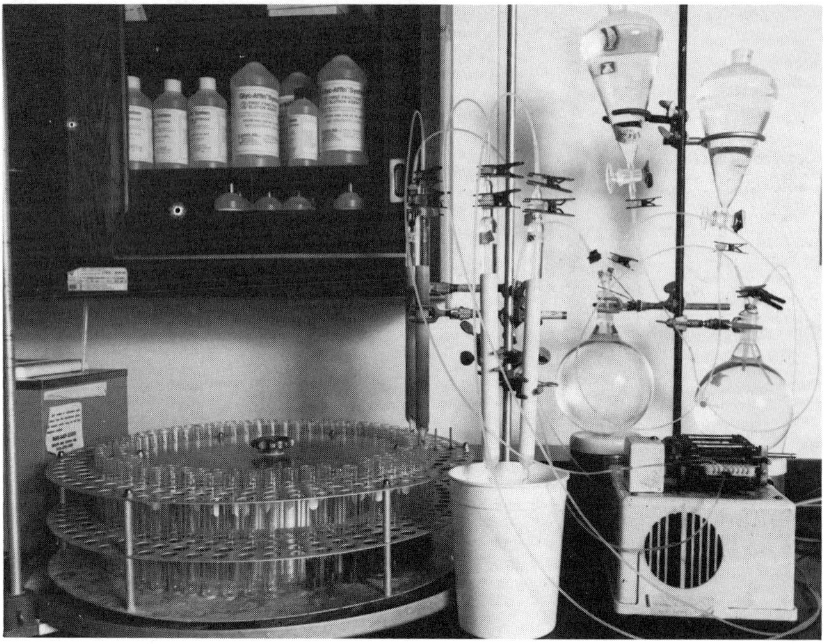

Figure 4.3 The basic units needed for a gradient-elution chromatographic system showing constant-volume mixing devices, separatory funnels, a pump, a fraction collector, and columns.

of the solutions—the smaller the mixer or the larger the difference between the molarities of the solutions, the steeper the gradient and vice versa. In another type of gradient device, solutions 1 and 2 are contained in two cylindrical vessels (Fig. 4.2) (4). Solution 1 of lower ionic strength is withdrawn and supplied to a column, while solution 2 enters solution 1 and mixes with it. Unlike the constant-volume device, the levels of liquid fall in both cylinders as chromatography continues, and both solutions are completely used up rather quickly, depending on the size of the cylinders. The type of the gradient will be linear throughout, and the magnitude of the gradient in the cylinder system depends upon the cross-sectional areas of the vessels and the concentrations of the buffers and their volume (usually the same for both the buffers). The greatest advantage of using the constant-volume mixing device is that the chromatography can be continued indefinitely, and several columns can be developed with one gradient device.

E. Macrochromatographic Separation and Quantitation of Glycosylated Hemoglobins

This can be achieved by gradient elution with developers containing sodium phosphate. Glycosylated Hbs in normal and diabetic adults (5), in various hemoglobinopathies with or without diabetes (3,6), and in newborn infants (2) are separated by applying a continuously increasing sodium phosphate gradient at a relatively constant pH (around pH 6.7). Developers 3-a, 6, 8, 9, and 10 with increasing phosphate concentrations with 0.019 to 0.3 M phosphate and pH varying between 6.75 and 6.50 (Table 4.1) are used. The gradients in all instances are made with constant-volume mixing devices. Depending upon the type of the gradient needed (shallow or steep), the size of the mixer can be chosen. The basic units needed for these chromatographic procedures are columns packed with the resin (homemade glass column will perform as well as commercially available ones), constant-volume mixing flask, separatory funnel for supplying developers of different molarities, pump for regulating the flow rate, fraction collector, uv/visible detector with a recorder (optional), and a temperature control for jacketed columns (optional). Figure 4.3 shows such a set-up. If a detector-recorder device is not used, the effluent fractions are read manually for heme absorbance in the Soret region (415 nm). The percentages of the Hb components are calculated on the basis of these absorbance readings.

Separation of Hb A_{Ia1}, Hb A_{Ia2}, Hb $A_{Ib1\text{-}3}$, Hb A_{Ic}, and Hb $A_{Id1\text{-}3}$ (see Fig. 3.2) in normal and diabetic adults is achieved by applying 250 mg of carbon monoxyhemoglobin to a 3 × 30 cm column of Bio-Rex 70 preequilibrated with Developer 6 and developing the column at 4°C (5). About 1 cm of the top of the resin layer is stirred, and the hemoglobin sample in Developer 6 is soaked in. A continuously increasing sodium phosphate gradient is obtained by supplying Developers 8 then 10 to a 1000-ml constant-volume mixing flask that contains Developer 6. A flow rate of 25 ml/hr is maintained, and 20-min fractions are collected. During the initial stage of the chromatographic development, Developer 8 is applied to the mixing flask until about 200 fractions are collected (Hb A_{Id3} will have been eluted by this time), after which Developer 8 is replaced by Developer 10. In addition to monitoring the absorbance at 415 nm, the first 20 fractions are also read at 280 nm to locate the nonheme protein peak.

Separation of Hb A_{Ia1}, Hb A_{Ia2}, Hb A_{Ib}, and Hb A_{Ic} also can be achieved using 0.05 M potassium phosphate, pH 6.60, as the starting buffer and utilizing a linear Na Cl gradient (7). Six grams of a red cell hemolysate are equilibrated with the starting buffer and loaded to a 5 × 40 cm column of Bio-Rex 70 equilibrated with at least 1 column volume of the starting buffer. A flow rate of 100 to 120 ml/hr is maintained, and 9-ml fractions are collected. After the elution of Hb A_{Ia1} and Hb A_{Ia2}, a linear gradient of 0.0 to 0.1 M NaCl in starting buffer (a total volume of 1000 ml in a two-cylinder device) is started. After the elution of Hb A_{Ib}, 0.1 M NaCl is con tinued until the Hb A_{Ic} peak is eluted. At this stage, the column is purged with 1 M NaCl to elute Hb A_o and Hb A_2 together.

The sodium phosphate gradient system described earlier is adaptable for the separation of glycosylated Hbs in various hemoglobinopathies (see Fig. 3.18) (3,6). Developers 6, 8, 9, and 10 are used with 2 × 25 cm and 1 × 25 cm columns of Bio-Rex 70 equilibrated with Developer 6 as the starting buffer. Thirty or 200 mg of Hb, depending upon the size of the column, are applied to the column and developed at room temperature. For a column 2 × 25 cm, a 1000-ml mixing flask is used, and for a column 1 × 25 cm a 500-ml flask is used to make the gradient. A sodium phosphate gradient is formed by supplying Developers 8, 9, and 10 in that order. A flow rate of 8-10 ml/hr is maintained for the smaller column and 16-18 ml/hr for the larger one; 20-min fractions are collected in both cases.

A slight modification of the sodium phosphate gradient applied for separation of the glycosylated hemoglobins in adult samples is necessary to achieve the separation of the glycosylated and acetylated minor fetal hemoglobin components in newborn infants or in adults with elevated levels of Hb F due to various hematologic disorders. With Developer 6 (0.038 M phosphate) as the starting buffer, Hb A_{Ic} will cochromatograph with Hb F_o, and Hb A_{Ia+b} with Hb $F_{I(s)}$. So, it is obvious that the molarity of the starting buffer has to be reduced so that Hb F and its minor components can be separated from adult major and minor hemoglobin components. Developer 3-a (0.019 M phosphate) has been introduced for this purpose (Table 4.1). Bio-Rex 70 resin is equilibrated initially in Developer 9, as discussed earlier, and subsequently equilibrated with Developer 3-a after packing the column. Thirty milligrams of hemolysate are dialyzed against Developer 3-a and applied to a 1 × 25 cm column. A 500-ml constant-volume mixing flask contains Developer 3-a, and a steadily increasing sodium phosphate gradient is formed by supplying Developer 6. After 24 hr, Developer 6 is replaced by

Developer 9. A flow rate of 12-15 ml/hr is maintained, and 20-min fractions are collected. Columns developed at room temperature are completed in 3-4 days. This chromatographic procedure separates the minor fetal hemoglobin components into Hb F_{Ia+b} and Hb F_{Ic} (see Fig. 3.10). For a complete separation of the minor fetal hemoglobin components to Hb F_{Ia1}, Hb F_{Ia2}, Hb F_{Ib}, and Hb F_{Ic} (see Fig. 3.11), a continuously increasing potassium phosphate gradient is utilized, and the columns are developed at 4°C (8). Developers 3-A, 6-A, 8-A, and 9-A, respectively, are 0.0135, 0.027, 0.054, and 0.108 M KH_2PO_4 containing no KCN, pH adjusted to 6.88 with 6 N KOH. Bio-Rex 70 is equiibrated with Developer 3-A, 30 mg Hb are applied to a 1 × 25 cm column, and 5-ml fractions are collected. One of the advantages with this system is not using KCN in the buffers. A similar potassium phosphate gradient, instead of a sodium phosphate gradient, also may be applied to separate adult minor hemoglobin components. However, with this system, the sample must be relatively fresh to avoid the presence of appreciable amounts of methemoglobin.

The gradient elution method for the separation of various Hb A_I's is cumbersome and time consuming if one is interested only in quantitating the minor fractions Hb A_{Ia+b} and Hb A_{Ic} in diabetics. Trivelli et al. (9) have developed a much faster approach to achieve this. Hb A_{Ia+b} and Hb A_{Ic} are eluted isocratically with Developer 6, followed by purging of the column with a high phosphate buffer (Developer 9) to elute the remaining hemoglobins. Different versions of the Trivelli procedure have been used by various laboratories without significantly affecting the separation of the minor Hb components. In one version, 30 mg of hemoglobin are applied to a 1 × 25 cm column of Bio-Rex 70 equilibrated with Developer 6 (10). The column is developed at room temperature initially with Developer 6 until Hb A_{Ia+b} and then Hb A_{Ic} are eluted, after which Developer 6 is replaced by Developer 9. A flow rate of 15 ml/hr is maintained, and 5-ml fractions are collected. The developers are supplied to the column directly without utilizing a gradient mixing device, thus a "stepwise gradient" system is utilized. Both Hb A_{Ia+b} and Hb A_{Ic} are readily separated. Figure 4.4 shows the separation of these minor hemoglobins in a normal adult and a diabetic patient. This method has been widely used for quantiatation of glycosylated hemoglobins in diabetic patients. In fact, many laboratories use this as a reference method for the levels of Hb A_{Ia+b} and Hb A_{Ic} or Hb A_{Ia+b+c} (Hb A_I). Moreover, this method has become the basis for the development of a variety of microchromatographic methods for quantitation of glycosylated hemoglobins.

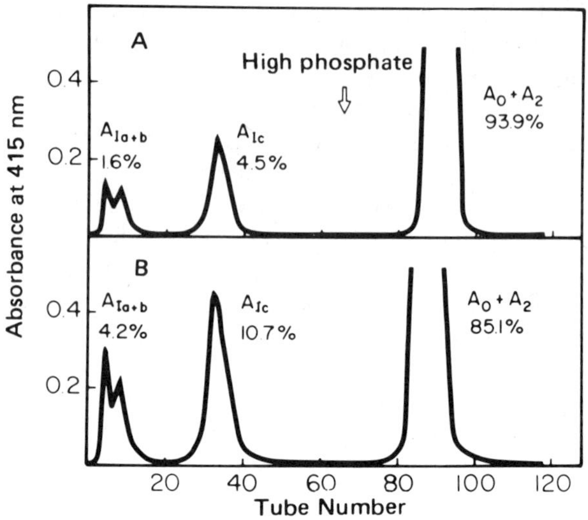

Figure 4.4 Bio-Rex 70 chromatographic separation of glycosylated components Hb A_{Ia+b} and Hb A_{Ic} according to Trivelli et al. (9) in a hemolysate from a normal control (A) and a diabetic patient (B). From Abraham et al. (10) by permission of the American Diabetes Association.

F. Microchromatographic Methods

A Survey of "Homemade" Microcolumn Methods

The concept of utilizing microcolumn chromatography for the separation and the quantitation of a specific hemoglobin is not quite new. For instance, anion exchange microchromatographic methods have been introduced about 10 years ago to quantitate Hb A_2 (11). With anion exchangers, such as DEAE-cellulose, under appropriate pH and molarity, Hb A_2 is eluted unretarded, whereas the other hemoglobins are retained by the column, which in turn can be stripped from the column. On the other hand, when cation exchangers are used, under appropriate conditions, Hb A_2 and Hb A_o are retained, while Hb $A_{I(s)}$ are eluted. During the last decade, various institutional and commercial laboratories have attempted to optimize the conditions for microchromatographic quantitation of Hb A_{Ia+b} and Hb A_{Ic} or just Hb A_{Ia+b+c} (Hb A_I). In general, the microchromatographic methods, because of their potential clinical application, have undergone extensive evaluation by comparing them with other well-established methods, such as the Trivelli, HPLC, and chemical methods, and ultimately by assessing the suitability of the micromethods for monitoring control of diabetes.

Kynoch and Lehman (12) first reported a short column method to quantitate Hb A_I. In this method, Bio-Rex 70 resin preequilibrated with a buffer (I) similar to Developer 6 is used to pack a 5-cm high column in 20-ml syringe barrel (2-cm internal diameter) with a small cotton plug at the bottom. The column is equilibrated by passing 50 ml of the buffer I through it. Anticoagulated blood (0.5 ml) is hymolyzed by a hemolyzing agent containing saponin, and the lysate is diluted with the starting buffer before applying to the top of the column. Hemoglobin A_I fraction is eluted with 100 ml of solution I, and the remainder of the hemoglobin (Hb A_o + Hb A_2) is eluted with solution II (similar to Developer 9). Chromatography is complete in 2½ hr. The absorbances of the fractions are determined at 413 nm, and the percantage of each fraction is determined on the basis of these readings. This methodology provides Hb A_I values in normal controls (6-9%) and in diabetics (6-19%) comparable to those obtained by conventional methods.

According to Jones et al. (13), microcolumns can be made by packing 8-cm long columns of Bio-Rex 70 in 5¾ in. disposable Pasteur pipettes. A plug of cotton at the constriction of each Pasteur pipette serves as the support for the resin. A 100-ml plastic funnel is attached to each column by means of a 7-cm length of rubber tubing. The column with the funnel is supported by a wooden rack that can hold six or more columns. Each column is equilibrated at room temperature using 40 ml of Developer 6. Three drops of a red cell hemolysate (11-12 g Hb/dl) are diluted with 9 drops of Developer 6 and applied to the column after it is detached from the funnel. Before sample application, resin, to the depth of 0.5 cm, is stirred together with 0.5 cm of the buffer above the column so that the sample can freely flow in and form a nice band of hemoglobin on the top. The funnel is attached to the column again, and the chromatography is initiated by adding 15-20 ml Developer 6 to the funnel. The effluent from the column is collected in three fractions, namely, Hb A_{Ia+b}, Hb A_{Ic}, and Hb A_o + Hb A_2, the division being made visually. Collection of Hb A_{Ia+b} is completed in the first 2.3-3.3 ml of the effluent in 25-35 min. Collection of Hb A_{Ic} is started then and continued for 90 min, during which time 4.5-6.5 ml may be collected. At this point, the major hemoglobin would be halfway down the column. The remainder of Developer 6 in the funnel is removed, and the high molarity buffer (Developer 9) is added to elute the remaining hemoglobins. The columns are ready for reuse after an overnight reequilibration with 40 ml of Developer 6. The percentages of the hemoglobin fractions are calculated on the basis of absorbance readings at

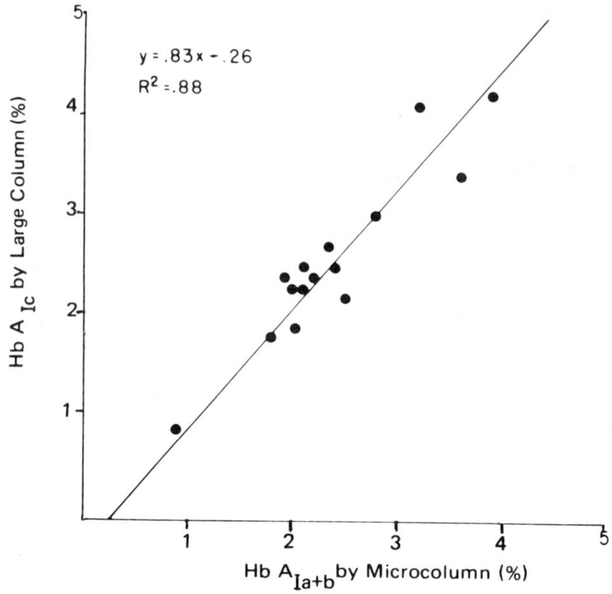

Figure 4.5 Correlation between the amounts of Hb A_{Ia+b} determined by the macrocolumn (large column) method of Trivelli et al. (9) and the microcolumn method of Jones et al. (13). Blood samples from 15 subjects including normals, one subject with hemolytic anemia, and diabetic patients were studied. Courtesy of Jones et al. (13).

415 nm. The percentages of Hb A_{Ia+b} and Hb A_{Ic} determined by this micromethod in normal and diabetic subjects correlated well with the values obtained by macrocolumn methodology (Figs. 4.5 and 4.6). Moreover, in about 3 hr, the minor hemoglobins can be determined with less expensive and complicated equipment. Obviously, one can modify this procedure by using a homemade manifold such as the one Efremov et al. (11) used for microquantitation of Hb A_2. With this modification, up to 20 samples can be run in a batch, the developers being supplied from one separatory funnel to all the columns. The reequilibration also can be made easier and faster by this approach.

Several modifications of the above microchromatographic procedure have appeared later. In one method, the separation on the Bio-Rex 70 resin is facilitated by introducing a 1-min centrifugation step (14). The device is composed of (a) a plastic container (28 × 80 mm) with a threaded top and a small vent

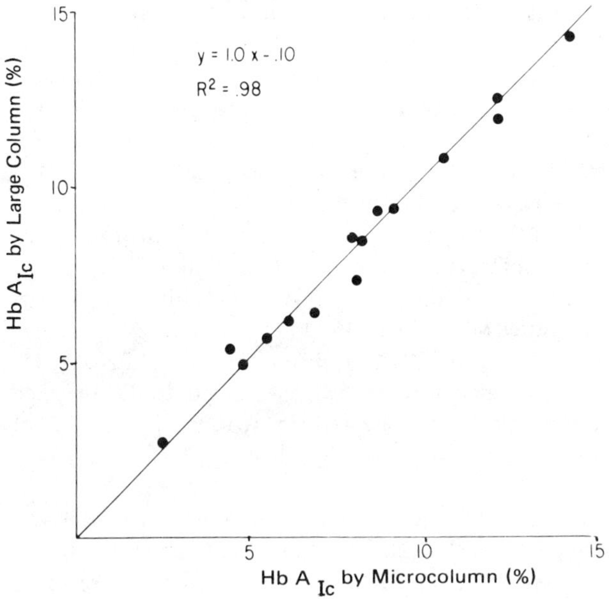

Figure 4.6 Correlation between the amounts of Hb A_{Ic} as determined by the large column method of Trivelli et al. (9) and by the microcolumn method of Jones et al. (13).

hole (1 mm) drilled approximately 3 mm below the threaded section and (b) a fluid reservoir and column section. After applying the sample, approximately 15 ml of buffer is added to the eluent reservoir, and the tubes are then centrifuged at 150-200 *g* for 1 min. The eluate (glycosylated Hb) is recovered from the lower reservoir. For total Hb determination, an aliquot of the original sample is diluted. The fastness of this method makes it an ideal means of assaying for Hb A_I in an out-patient clinic setup. The "minicolumn" used in this method can be filled with less than 2 g of ion exchanger, and only a small sample of blood is required.

In another technique (15), columns are packed in 20-ml syringe barrels, the tops of the columns being closed with rubber stoppers with No. 22 gauge needles. The needle point is bent upward so that the solution coming through the needle will not disturb the surface of the resin bed. Connect each of three columns to a Technicon three-way glass fitting. Connect the delivery end of the glass fitting to a three-way valve that can select the eluent from a reservoir. Deliver a 0.5-ml aliquot of hemolysate to the top of the column, open the valve under the column, and start collecting the eluate in a 100-ml volumetric flask. When the hemolysate is drained into the column, 4 ml of the elution buffer are added to the top of the resin bed. After closing the column with the stopper with the delivery needle, the valve connecting the reservoir with the elution buffer is opened to collect the Hb A_I fraction in the 100-ml volumetric flask, and the absorbance at 540 nm is determined. Instead of collecting the remaining hemoglobins, the absorbance of an aliquot of 0.5 ml hemolysate diluted to 100 ml is determined. Fifty-two male diabetic patients and 18 normal men were studied with this method (15). Coefficients of variation (CV) were 2.3% within run and 3.4% run to run. The level of Hb A_I in normals was 6.6 ± 1.4% and in diabetics 10.8 ± 2.5%. The data also revealed a relationship between fasting plasma glucose and Hb A_I values ($\gamma = 0.75$) only in normal or high-normal regions; however, at high glucose values, a plateau was approached.

Maquart et al. (16) modified the microcolumn methodology by continuously reading the effluent optical densities. A microcolumn with 0.6-cm internal diameter is connected through a Teflon capillary to the flow cell of a spectrophotometer equipped with a recorder, and the flow cell is connected to a pump. Red cell hemolysate equivalent to 7.5 mg Hb is applied to a 12-cm column and developed with a flow rate of 0.32 ml/min, and the elution is monitored by recording the optical density at 415 nm. Two fractions, Hb A_{Ia+b} and Hb A_{Ic}, are collected. Sixteen normal subjects and 32 diabetic patients were studied with this method. The mean percentage of Hb A_{Ic} in the normals was 5.0% (3.2-6.1%), in poorly treated diabetic patients 8.9% (5.5-15.3%), and in rather well-controlled patients 6.4% (5.7%-7.1%).

Automation of micro- or macrochromatographic techniques was the goal of some laboratories. Two automated techniques have been reported (17,18). In one system, automation is achieved by adapting an automatic peptide analyzer (17). A three-buffer system enables complete and rapid peak separations of Hb A_{Ia+b}, Hb A_{Ic}, and Hb A_o. Up to 200 samples can be analyzed in 1 week. Automation of chromatographic separations is also achieved by adapting a single column amino acid analyzer for separation of hemoglobins by Bio-Rex 70 resin and monitoring the absorbance at a wavelength of 570 nm (18). The separation of Hb A_{Ia+b} from Hb A_{Ic} is incomplete but both fractions are widely separated from Hb A_o. This procedure can be completed in 45 min with reasonable precision and reproducibility.

An Improved Microcolumn Method for Quantitation of Hb A_{Ia+b} and Hb A_{Ic}

As will be discussed later in this section, cation exchange microchromatography is subject to interferences by variation in temperature and by the presence of the aldimine Schiff base. Also, using KCN-containing buffers may not be generally acceptable. To circumvent these problems, a modified microcolumn method was developed in our laboratory (Bissé and Abraham, unpublished information). This method utilizes Bio-Rex 70 resin and developers containing both sodium phosphate and potassium phosphate and also NaCl, but no KCN. The chromatograms are developed at a column pH of around 6.3, which is close to the pK of the carboxylic groups of Bio-Rex 70 resin. This approach improves the buffering action and reduces the particle size of the resin.

Mainly, three developers are needed for this method. Developer 1 contains 54.8 mmol/liter $NaH_2PO_4 \cdot H_2O$, 13.8 mmol/liter Na_2HPO_4, and 8.55 mmol/liter NaCl. Developer 2 contains 54.8 mmol/liter $NaH_2PO_4 \cdot H_2O$, 13.8 mmol/liter Na_2HPO_4, and 41 mmol/liter NaCl. The pH of both the developers is adjusted to 6.5 with a potassium phosphate solution (34.84 g/liter K_2HPO_4 and 79.9 g/liter $K_3PO_4 \cdot 3H_2O$). The final ionic strength of Developer 1 and Developer 2 expressed as Siemens and measured in a conductometer are 5 and 7, respectively. Developer 3 is a solution of 0.6 M NaCl.

Thirty grams of Bio-Rex 70 were dispersed in 400 ml of distilled warer and degassed for 15 min under vacuum. The supernatant is discarded and resuspended again in 400 ml of water. The pH of the resin suspension is adjusted to 6.1 with concentrated phosphoric acid with thorough stirring. The resin in settled, water is discarded, and reequilibration is done in Developer 1 until a pH of 6.38 is attained. A 50% suspension is transferred into a 7 mm × 8.5 cm column (which includes a wide top of about 2.5 cm length that served as a reservoir for the developer) until the packed resin reaches 4.5 cm. (This requires about 1.8 g of the slurry.) Empty plastic columns for packing such columns are available from various commercial sources. A porous polyethylene disc placed at the bottom of the column serves as the support for the resin. Another porous disc may be placed above the gel surface, although this step is not highly essential. The microcolumn may be packed in regular Pasteur pipettes with a funnel attachment used for holding the developer.

Blood, collected in ethylenediaminetetraacetic acid (EDTA)-containing tubes, is centrifuged to remove the plasma. One volume of packed cells is mixed with an equal volume of distilled water followed by vigorous vortexing for achieving complete lysis. To dissociate the aldimine Schiff base, the hemolysate is diluted with 1.5 volumes of 0.05 M potassium biphthalate, pH 5.0, and is incubated at 37°C for 15 min. The diluted hemolysate is then centrifuged to settle the remaining proteins precipitated by lowering the pH of the sample.

A 50-μl hemolysate (about 2.5 mg Hb) prepared as described above is applied to the top of the microcolumn and allowed to soak in. The sample is washed down into the resin with 100 μl of Developer 2. The Hb A_{Ia+b} fraction is collected by passing 1.8 ml of Developer 2 through the column. The second fraction, containing Hb A_{Ic}, is then eluted with 2 ml of the same developer. Finally, the remaining Hbs are eluted with 2 ml of Developer 3 and diluted by adding 20 ml of distilled water. The absorbance of the fractions is read at 415 nm, and the percentages of Hb A_{Ia+b} and Hb A_{Ic} are calculated in the following manner:

$$\%\ \text{Hb}\ A_{Ia+b} = \frac{0.85x \times 100}{0.85\ x + y + 11z}$$

$$\%\ \text{Hb}\ A_{Ic} = \frac{y \times 100}{0.85x + y + 11z}$$

where x, y, and z are the absorbances of Hb A_{Ia+b}, Hb A_{Ic}, and Hb A_o, respectively.

This microchromatographic methodology has undergone evaluation by correlating the Hb A_{Ia+b} and Hb A_{Ic} values obtained by this new method with the values obtained by HPLC and by conventional Bio-Rex 70 machrochromatography (Figs. 4.7 and 4.8). Correlations of Hb A_{Ic} values by the new micromethod with the values obtained by the macromethod and by the HPLC technique were excellent. Likewise, Hb A_{Ia+b} values obtained by the micromethod correlated well with the values obtained by the macromethod. However, the correlation was decidedly poor when the Hb A_{Ia+b} values of the micromethod and the HPLC method were compared. It is apparent that Bio-Rex 70 cation exchange chromatographic techniques give higher values for Hb A_{Ia+b} than the HPLC method. The intraassay CV was 2.5 and 3% for normal and diabetic samples, respectively, whereas the interassay CV was 5.5 and 5%.

The effect of the temperature on the column was studied between 20° and 35°C, using both normal and diabetic samples. Fluctuation in temperature from 20 to 30°C produced no significant changes in the values obtained for Hb

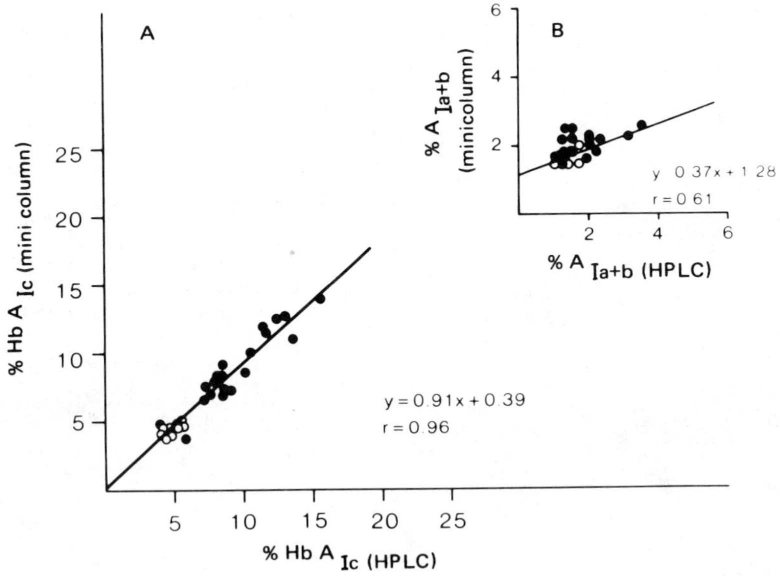

Figure 4.7 Correlation between the Hb A_{Ic} (A) and Hb A_{Ia+b} (B) values determined by the new microchromatographic method ("minicolumn") of Bissé and by HPLC in normal controls (○) and in diabetic patients (●).

A_{Ic} (Fig. 4.9). The reason for this is presumably due to the fact that the chromatography in performed near the pK of the cation exchanger. Raising the temperature above 30°C increased the Hb A_{Ic} values more than 10% compared to the values at 20°C. To determine the efficiency of the new procedure to remove the Schiff base during the sample preparation, erythrocytes from normal subjects were incubated with various concentrations of glucose, and the total Hb A_I was determined by the new method and also by the Isolab Fast Hemoglobin System (no aldimine elimination step was used with the Isolab method). The results clearly indicated that the sample preparation technique used in the new method eliminates all the aldimine, and thus only the ketoamine form of the glycosylated Hbs is quantitated.

Commercially Available Microcolumn Methods

Several short-column methods employing disposable columns and resin are now commercially available to quantitate total Hb A_I or Hb A_{Ia+b} and Hb A_{Ic}.

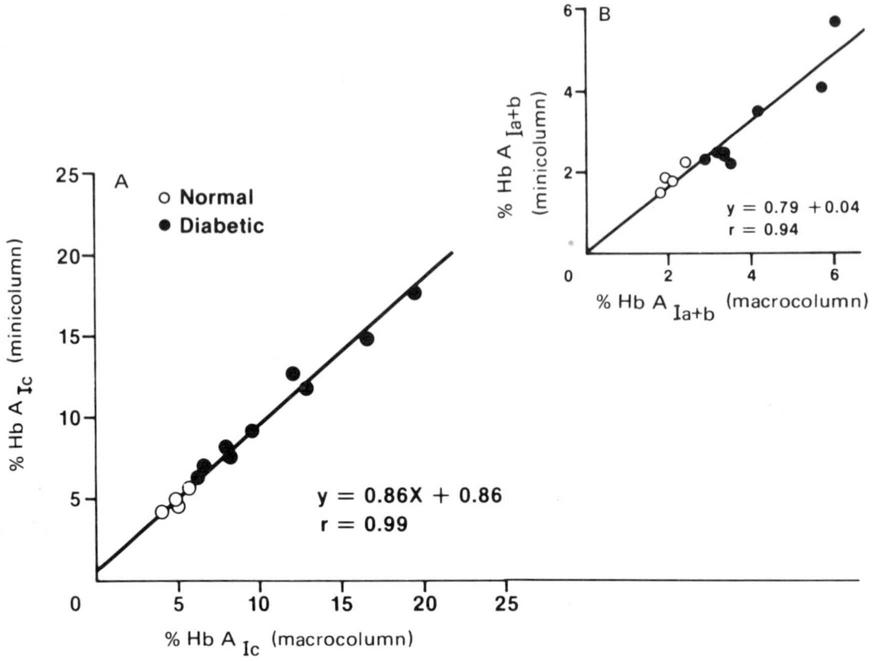

Figure 4.8 Correlation between the values of Hb A_{Ic} (A) and Hb A_{Ia+b} (B) as determined by the new microchromatographic method of Bissé and Abraham and by the classical Trivelli method.

separately. One such column, which we have had considerable experience with, is made by Isolab, Inc. (Akron, Ohio) (10). These are obtainable under the trade name Quik-Sep Fast Hemoglobin Test System. These are plastic columns about 8.5 cm (total length) with about 2.5 X 2 cm reservoir for the buffer at the top (Fig. 4.10). The actual usable part of the column is about 7 mm X 6 cm. A porous polyethylene disc is placed at the bottom, and another disc 0.5 cm above the gel surface of a 4.5 cm long column. The packing material, IRC-50 or Bio-Rex 70, is suspended in a buffer similar to Developer 6, but made with potassium phosphate and containing sodium azide. The columns are transported after the top and the bottom are capped air-tight to prevent leaking of the buffer. The company also supplies a sample preparation reagent, the solutions necessary for developing the columns, and a set of Fast Hemoglobin

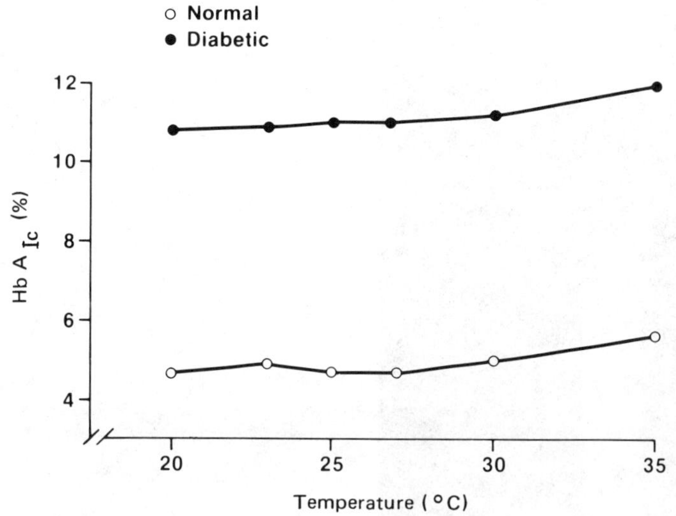

Figure 4.9 Temperature dependence of Hb A_{Ic} determined by the method of Bissé in a normal and a diabetic person.

Control. Similar microchromatographic systems may be obtained from other commercial sources, such as Helena Laboratories (Beaumont, Texas), Bio-Rad Laboratories (Richmond, Calif.), Sigma Chemical Co. (St. Louis, Mo.), and perhaps other sources as well.

One of the commercial microcolumn methods that has undergone extensive evaluation in our hands is the Isolab Quik-Sep Fast Hemoglobin System (10). The sample preparation and the chromatographic steps for this method are as follows (*Informational Bulletin,* Isolab, Ind.): Whole blood sample (50 μl) is hemolyzed with the Fast Hemoglobin Sample Preparation Reagent (200 μl) by occasional shaking for 10 min. Freshly drawn blood samples with EDTA as the anticoagulant or samples preserved at 4°C are used. Considerable fluctuation in the levels of Hb A_I can occur due to the presence of variable amounts of the aldmine Schiff base (this aspect will be later discussed in more detail) in diabetic patients, thus leading to misinterpretation of the results. The aldimine can be eliminated before applying the sample to the column by lysing the blood sample with the Fast Hb Aldimine Eliminator (supplied by the same company) in place of the sample preparation reagent. Mix 50 μl of blood with 200 μl of Aldimine Eliminator. Shake and let stand

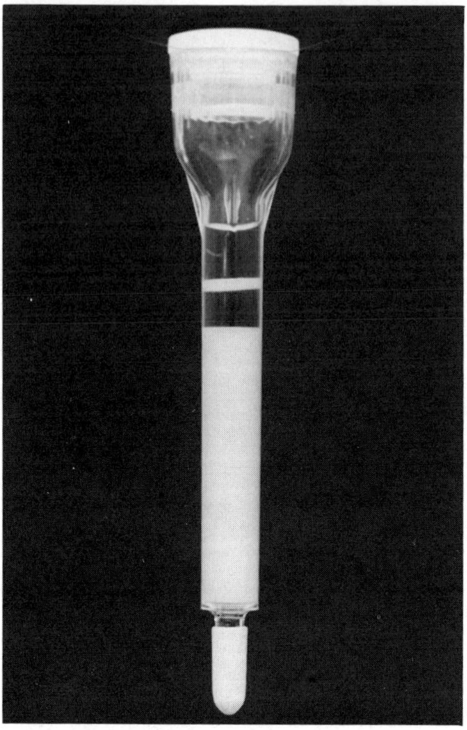

Figure 4.10 Quik-Sep Fast Hemoglobin Column (Isolab Inc., Akron, Ohio).

for 60 min at room temperature with occasional shaking, or mix as above and incubate at 37°C for 20 min. The Aldimine Eliminator is an adicified surfactant solution that lyses the red cells, and the low pH favors the dissociation of the Schiff base. A fresh Quik-Sep column is used each time. For preparation of the column, remove the top cap first and then the bottom closure; this order of opening is important to avoid air entering from the tip. After the column has started to drain, push the top disc down until it contacts the top of the gel bed. Add 50 μl of the hemolysate to the top of the column. Allow the column to drain until the liquid level reaches the top disc. Add 4 ml of Fast Hb Elution Solutions (Solution No. 1) to the top of the column and collect the fast hemoglobin (Hb A_I) fraction. The elution will stop when the liquid level reaches the top disc. This step will take less than 30 min. The other hemoglobin that is retained on the column is eluted with 4 ml of the Elution Agent: Other Hemoglobin (Solution No. 2). The other hemoglobin fraction is diluted with 16 ml of water, and the Fast Hemoglobin fraction is undiluted before reading the optical density at 415 nm. If A is the absorbance of the fast hemoglobin (Hb A_I) and H is the absorbance of the other hemoglobins, then

$$\% \text{ Hb } A_I = \frac{A \times 100}{A + 5H}$$

If the column is loaded with the necessary amounts of Hb: A ranges from 0.1 to 0.3 and H ranges from 0.4 to 0.8. Instead of eluting the other hemoglobin fraction, the absorbance of the total Hb (Hb A_I + other hemoglobin) may be determined by diluting a 50-μl aliquot of the hemolysate with 16 ml of water and 4 ml of the Other Hemoglobin Elution Agent. This approach will save about 20 min of analysis time.

The influence of ambient temperature on Hb A_I values determined by these microcolumns has been well documented (19,20). In fact, there is a direct correlation between the column temperature and Hb A_I values. Since ambient temperature is bound to fluctuate, the reproducibility of Hb A_I determination can be easily affected. One can approach this problem in two ways. One way is to perform the chromatography at 23° ± 0.1°C in a temperature-controlled device. Water from a circulating water bath flows through a plexiglass-jacketed device which can accommodate up to 20 microcolumns. Alternatively, the ambient temperature at which the chromatography is done is recorded, and the Hb A_I values are corrected to results at 23°C utilizing a temperature correction table supplied by the column manufacturer or prepared in the user's laboratory. Correction for temperature effect was more closely looked into, and noteworthy results have been reported (21). The CV for Hb A_I of the samples run with a temperature-controlled system ranged from 1.8 to 4.5%, whereas the CV for the ambient run corrected values ranged from 9.5 to 18%. The mean ambient run corrected values for Hb A_I were consistently lower than the values for samples run when temperature was regulated at 23°C. It is also important that a set of lyophilized controls are run with the samples. Such controls are commercially available or "in-house" freeze-dried controls may be used (22). Ideally, a normal, medium high, and a high Hb A_I control should be included.

Hemoglobin A_I values determined by this microcolumn method correlated very well with the Hb A_{Ic} and Hb A_I values determined by HPLC on Synchropak CM 300 cation exchange columns (Figs. 4.11 and 4.12). The

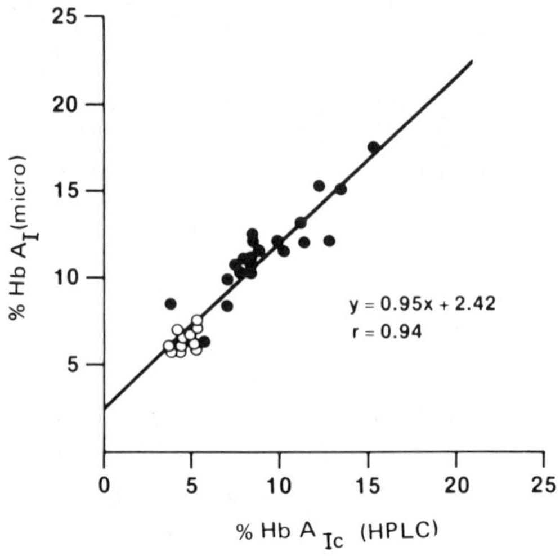

Figure 4.11 Correlation of Hb A_I levels determined by the Isolab Quik-Sep Fast Hemoglobin method with the Hb A_{Ic} levels determined by HPLC on Synchropak CM 300 column in normal controls (○) and diabetic patients (●).

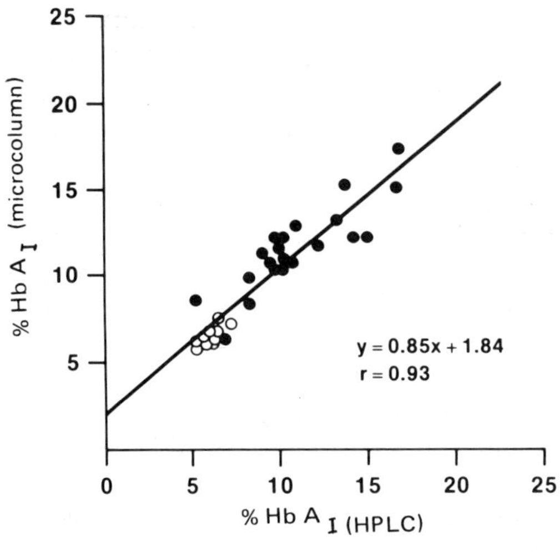

Figure 4.12 Correlation of Hb A_I levels determined by the Isolab Quik-Sep Fast Hemoglobin method with the Hb A_I (Hb A_{Ia+b+c}) levels determined by HPLC on Synchropak CM 300 column in normal controls (○) and diabetic patients (●).

microchromatographic methodology for Hb A_I determinations gave good precision and reproducibility as depicted by CV of 0.5-0.8% within run and 1.0-2.2% between run. The normal levels of Hb A_I obtained in our laboratory with the Isolab microcolumns are 6.0 ± 0.8% (4.2-7.6%), and the levels in diabetics are 13.0 ± 2.6% (9.4-18.9%).

As mentioned earlier, several companies are making cation exchange microcolumns. This author does not particularly recommend columns from one manufacturer or the other. However, it is worth mentioning that in an evaluation of three commercially available microcolumns (Isolab, Helena, and Bio-Rad), by correlating the Hb A_I values with Hb A_{Ic} levels determined by an HPLC method in 121 samples from diabetic patients, the Isolab method showed the highest correlation (23). Ths Isolab and the Helena methods gave results that were linear with percentages of Hb A_I as high as 30%. The results by the Bio-Rad method, on the other hand, were slightly nonlinear at values over 15%. The Isolab method also showed better precision (CV) within and between assays than the other two methods.

G. Factors Influencing Glycosylated Hemoglobin Determination by Cation Exchange Chromatography

pH, Molarity, and Temperature

Several laboratories have attempted to optimize the conditions for measurement of glycosylated Hbs with cation exchange columns, microcolumns in particular. From a practical standpoint, chromatographic conditions, such as pH, phosphate buffer concentration, and temperature, are three important factors having great influence on the chromatographic separation and the glycosylated hemoglobin level; these critical factors have been looked into in great detail (20,24). At pH 6.72, it seems that nearly complete recovery of Hb A_{Ic} is obtained with very little Hb A_o contamination. The elution depends strongly on pH, and the pH tolerance of the buffer is less than 0.05 pH units. Above pH 6.8 there is a steep increase in fast hemoglobin levels. The phosphate molarity of the elution is also highly critical. At 0.025 M, little hemoglobin is eluted, while at 0.1-0.15 M, almost all hemoglobin fractions are eluted. A combination of equilibration and elution buffer molarities would provide full recovery of the Hb A_{Ic} peak. Yet another laboratory has reported an optimum pH of 6.85 and buffer concentrations of 87 mOsm/kg (24). Separation is also good at pH 6.8 and a buffer concentration of 97 mOsm/kg. However, at pH 6.8 and a buffer concentration 87 mOsm/kg, some of the Hb A_I is

Table 4.2 Fast Hb and pH at Selected Temperatures

Temperature (°C)	Fast Hb (%)	Buffer pH	Resin pH
16	3.70	6.77	6.72
19	5.86	6.78	6.76
20	6.68	6.79	6.77
21	6.96	6.79	6.78
22	8.23	6.80	6.79
23	8.62	6.80	6.80
24	8.62	6.81	6.81
25	9.20	6.81	6.82
26	9.76	6.82	6.83
27	10.72	6.82	6.84
30	12.98	6.84	6.87
35	23.85	6.86	6.91

Source: From Rosenthal (19).

retained on the column, whereas at 6.85 pH and 97 mOsm/kg, some of Hb A_0 is eluted with Hb A_I. Thus, it is obvious that while using "homemade" columns and developers, each laboratory has to work out their own optimum conditions for the separation of glycosylated Hbs in micro- or even macrochromatography.

The chromatographic property of hemoglobin on Bio-Rex 70 resin are temperature dependent (19,20,25,26). This seems to be the result of differential rates of exchange and affinities for charged molecules by ion-exchange resins as a function of temperature. Thus, the separations on the weak carboxylate cation exchange resin, microchromatographic separations in particular, can be greatly influenced by variations in ambient temperature. When the effect of temperature on a microcolumn method was evaluated, noteworthy results were obtained (19,26). As shown in Table 4.2, with increasing pH, There was an increase in the levels of Hb A_I. There was also a direct relationship between pH and the percent of fast hemoglobin (Hb A_I) at varying temperatures. The effect of temperature appears to be partly due to its effect on buffer and resin pHs. The optimum temperature for the fast Hb assay is 22°-24°C. In this region, the microcolumn values are the closest to the control values as determined by a reference method. So, it is highly recommended that the temperature in the test area be monitored when the determinations are performed, the test be run between 22° and 24°C, and the measured percentage of glycosylated Hb be converted to values at 23°C using a temperature correction chart. Using a temperature-controlled device is another alternative.

Labile Schiff Base (Pre-Hb A_{Ic})

The formation of glycosylated hemoglobin proceeds through the initial rapid formation of the labile aldimine or Schiff base (pre-A_{Ic}) that can subsequently undergo Amadori rearrangement forming the stabile ketoamine. Most conventional chromatographic and electrophoretic methods do not distinguish the labile form from the stable form, and both are separated as a single entity. Inclusion of the labile form with the stable form can lead to overestimation of glycosylated hemoglobin levels, thus weakening the reliability of using Hb A_{Ic} (or Hb A_I) values for chronic glucose control.

Various laboratories have used both in vivo and in vitro studies to demonstrate rapid changes in chromatographically determined Hb A_{Ic} or Hb A_I induced by short-term changes in glucose concentrations (26-32). In vitro at 37°C, chromatographically determined Hb A_{Ic} (contains both stable and labile types) increased with glucose concentration and time in erythrocytes from normal and diabetic persons (29). When incubated with 20-100 mM glucose, the increase in Hb A_{Ic} was maximal at 4-6 hr and then stayed unchanged for the next 18-20 hr. After a rapidly produced increase, Hb A_{Ic} decreased to the preincubation level during a further incubation of the erythrocytes in a glucose-free medium for another 4-6 hr. The linear increase with time of Hb A_{Ic} was about 0.034% hr^{-1} mmol/liter glucose and the linear decrease was 0.017% hr^{-1} mmol/liter glucose. Incubation of red cells with high concentration of glucose (up to 100 mM) for 24 hr produced only 1.3% of stable Hb A_{Ic}. Chemical analysis (TBA assay) of the hemoglobin after incubation with high concentration of glucose supported the concept that the formation of the labile aldimine is favored under these conditions. In vivo evidence also points to a mechanism by which short-term increases or decreases in glucose concentration can respond to corresponding changes in Hb A_{Ic} through the formation of, or the dissociation of, the labile aldimine. For instance, in juvenile diabetic patients undergoing treatment, rapid changes of blood glucose concentration of up to 20 mmol/liter resulted in an increase in Hb A_{Ic} concentration of 1.9% within 12 hr (29). Such changes were reversible by normalization of the glucose level. Direct demonstration of changes in the levels of labile Schiff base is possible only if this pre-Hb A_{Ic} can be separated from Hb A_{Ic}. Separation of

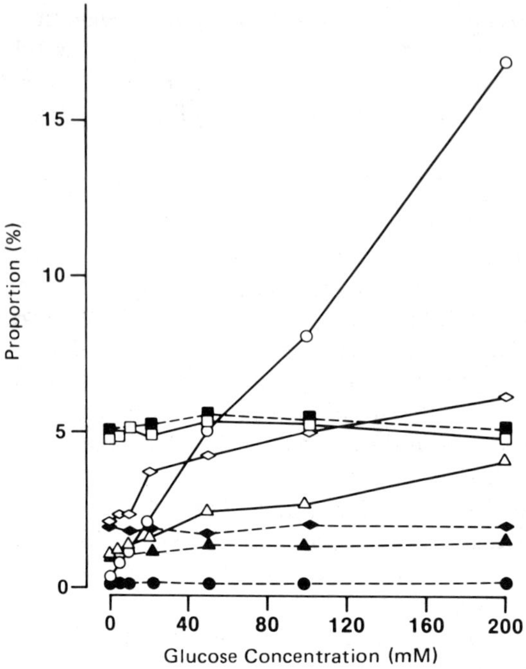

Figure 4.13 Proportion of the minor components Hb A_{Ia+b} (△), pre-Hb A_{Ic} (○), Hb A_{Ic} (□), and Hb A_{Id} (◇) in red cells after incubation with 0-200 mM glucose as determined by cation exchange HPLC. The dashed lines and the closed symbols represent the corresponding values after elimination of the aldimine by treatment with 0.05 M potassium bipthalate, pH 5.0. From Stallings and Abraham (32).

the labile Schiff base from the ketoamine was, in fact, achieved by Mortensen (30,31) utilizing isoelectric focusing and by Stallings and Abraham (32) with HPLC. With the application of these methods, a direct correlation between glucose levels and concentration of the labile intermediate was shown (30,32). Moreover, during one of these studies (32), a linear increase in the labile forms of Hb A_{Ia+b}, Hb A_{Ic}, and Hb A_{Id} with increasing glucose concentration was documented (Fig. 4.13). However, during a 3-hr incubation with glucose (0 to 200 mM), no increase in the stable forms of these minor Hb components was observed. The importance of eliminating the labile aldimine and measuring only the stabile ketoamine was emphasized by Compagnucci et al. (33) because of the observation that day-to-day variation in stable Hb A_I was absent in both stable and unstable diabetics (33). The authors concluded that significant fluctuations in total Hb A_I reduce its value as an index of long-term control in unstable diabetics, while a single determination of Hb A_I closely reflects blood glucose control over the previous 2 months. Moreover, according to Mortensen (30), in postprandial blood samples (1-5 hr after a meal), changes in blood glucose concentration were followed by corresponding changes in the percentages of pre-A_{Ic}, while Hb A_{Ic} remained unchanged. Plasma glucose levels correlated with simultaneously determined total and labile Hb A_I fractions, but not with stable Hb A_I. In subjects with impaired oral glucose tolerance, similar changes in total, but not in stable, Hb A_I were obtained during glucose tolerance test. Thus, it seems that to ensure more accurate index of blood long-term glucose control, measurement of stable glycosylated hemoglobin A_I needs to be performed.

Several methods have been proposed, and some have been routinely used to eliminate the aldimine from red cell hemolysate before the chromatographic step. One of the simplest, yet time-consuming, means of achieving this is to incubate red cells in 100 volumes of isotonic saline for 6 hr at 37°C. In this method, the concentration of stable Hb A_I is defined as the concentration that is chromatographically determined after an incubation of RBC in glucose-free solution for 6 hr at 37°C. The concentration of the labile Hb A_I is the difference between the concentration of Hb A_I obtained before and after the incubation of RBC in glucose-free solution. The other obvious and relatively simple method would be to prepare the hemolysate first and then dialyze against 1000 volumes of the buffer. Pressure filtration of the hemolysate has been successfully used to eliminate the aldimine. In a rapid chemical method for aldimine elimination, red cells are incubated for 30 min at 37°C with 30 mM semicarbazide and 12 mM aniline, pH 5.0 (34). After the incubation, the red cells are centrifuged, the supernatant is aspirated, and the packed cells are prepared for assay. Yet another method simply utilizes lysing of the red cells with 0.05 M potassium bipthalate buffer, pH 5.0, making use of the instability of the Schiff base adduct in acidic solution (35). At this pH, dissociation of the Schiff base reaches completion during sample preparation.

Fetal and Abnormal Hemoglobins

Hemoglobin F cochromatographs with Hb A_{Ic} on Bio-Rex 70 cation exchange macro- or microcolumns and thus interferes with the quantitation of this minor hemoglobin. This chromatographic approach is not apparently suitable for quantitation of Hb A_{Ic} (or Hb A_I) in blood samples containing elevated levels of Hb F, i.e., blood from newborn infants, pregnant women, patients with chronic myelogenous leukemia, and patients with various hemoglobinopathies. Accurate quantitation of Hb A_{Ic} or Hb A_I in the presence of Hb F requires an independent estimate of the amounts of Hb F or a method that is not affected by Hb F, such as affinity chromatography, isoelectric focusing, radioimmunoassay, and some chemical methods (these methods will be discussed later in this section).

The pressure of faster or slower moving hemoglobin variants will greatly influence the levels of Hb A_I determined by cation exchange chromatography (3,6,36-42). Like Hb F, fast-moving hemoglobin H (β_4) in α-thalassemic patients, N-Baltimore ($\alpha_2\beta_2{}^{95\ \mathrm{Lys}\rightarrow\mathrm{Glu}}$), and J-Baltimore ($\alpha_2\beta_2{}^{16\ \mathrm{Gly}\rightarrow\mathrm{Asp}}$) may interfere with Hb A_I quantitation. The presence of these hemoglobins will produce an apparent increase in the levels of Hb A_I because these Hbs may co-elute with Hb A_I. Slow-moving hemoglobins S, C, D, and E, on the other hand, cause an apparent lowering of Hb A_I levels determined by cation exchange microchromatography. This is simply because the glycosylated counterparts of these abnormal hemoglobins are retained by the ion exchange column after Hb A_I is eluted. However, it should be pointed out that, as discussed earlier in this section, it is possible to separate the glycosylated forms of the normal Hb and the slow-moving abnormal hemoglobins with cation exchange macrochromatography or by HPLC.

Acetylation by Aspirin

Aspirin (acetylsalicylic acid) modifies several sites, presumably lysines, on both the α and β chains of Hb A (43-45). Acetylation of lysine residues with aspirin confers a negative charge on the modified protein. The modified hemoglobin has altered electrophoretic and chromatographic properties. It also migrates ahead of Hb A_o, like Hb A_I, on CM-cellulose or HPLC cation exchange columns. Patients on long-term high-dose aspirin therapy have a twofold increase in the modified hemoglobin. Also, a linear increase in Hb A_I has been demonstrated with increasing aspirin concentration and time of incubation of red cells, hemolysate, or purified Hb A_o. Thus, it is not surprising that patients receiving high doses of aspirin have increased levels of Hb A_I-like hemoglobins.

Carbamylation in Uremia

Elevated levels of both total Hb A_I- and Hb A_{Ic}-like hemoglobins have been reported in patients having uremia due to renal failure (46-51). In renal failure, most patients also have impaired glucose tolerance, and those on chronic dialysis are usually dialyzed against fluid with a high glucose content. So, it is likely that some of the increase in Hb A_I is due to the presence of increased glycosylated hemoglobins. However, colorimetric estimate of the glycosylated hemoglobin does not show such an increase in uremic patients. It now appears that most of the increase in fast hemoglobins in uremic patients are due to carbamylation of hemoglobin with cyanate, a consequence of the spontaneous dissociation of urea into cyanate and ammonia. Cyanate seems to react with protein amino groups, preferentially but not exclusively with α-amino groups. Flückiger et al. (51) determined the levels of altered hemoglobins in 14 renal patients. The levels of Hb A_I in these patients, as determined by Bio-Rex 70 column chromatography, increased from an average of 7.12% in the control group to 8.79% in the dialyzed group and 10.78% in the stable uremic group. The increase in Hb A_I was due entirely to an increase in the Hb A_{Ia+b} fraction, and the levels correlated significantly with predialysis blood urea nitrogen levels. In vitro carbamylation also produced carbamylated hemoglobin that eluted with Hb A_{Ia+b}. It should be pointed out that interpretation of the levels of glycosylated hemoglobin in uremia is complicated by the presence of anemia, even when chemical means are used to assay for glycosylated hemoglobin. Certainly, Hb A_I determinations by ion exchange methods in uremic patients should be interpreted with caution.

Modification by Acetaldehyde

People abusing alcohol have elevated levels of minor hemoglobins (Hb A_I), but yet are not diabetic (52). The levels of Hb A_{Ic}, as determined by radioimmunoassay, are normal in these persons. Acetaldehyde, a primary metabolite of ethanol, is present in the blood of these people at a concentration of 1-50 μmol/liter or even higher in persons chronically abusing alcohol. The increase in the minor hemoglobin is apparently due to formation of stable adducts between hemoglobins and acetaldehyde or 5-deoxy-D-xylulose 1-phosphate, an endogenous condensation product of acetaldehyde and dihydroxyacetone phosphate. At physiologic concentrations of acetaldehyde, stable adducts are also formed in vitro (52-54). The modified hemoglobins formed in this manner produce chromatographic variants, some of which migrate in the Hb $A_{Ia\text{-}c}$ region. Thus, alcoholics can be misinterpreted as having diabetes, on the basis of Hb A_I values. Analysis of stable adducts demonstrated that valine, lysine, and tyrosine residues of globin are sites of reaction. This may be the reason why up to five hemoglobin-acetaldehyde adducts have been noticed with Bio-Rex 70 and high-pressure liquid chromatographic methods (52-55).

Hyperlipidemia or Lactescence

When whole blood samples are used for quantitation of Hb A_I, lactescent plasma due to hyperlipoproteinemia can cause false elevation of Hb A_I. This is simply due to the fact that lactescence elutes in the first (Hb A_I) fraction and absorb at 415 nm. According to Dix et al. (56), the apparent Hb A_I in a nondiabetic person with type V hyperlipoproteinemia with a plasma triglyceride concentration of 40 g/liter was 11.9% when whole blood sample was analyzed (56). In a hemolysate prepared from washed cells free of plasma, Hb A_I was substantially less (7.5%). This difference of 4.4% is attributable to lactescence in the plasma. When cell-free plasma was applied to a column, all the lactescence (measured by A_{415}) appeared in the first fraction (Hb A_I). Blood specimens containing various concentrations of triglycerides from diabetic patients were used to quantitate glycosylated hemoglobins by ion exchange microcolumn chromatography and by agar gel electrophoresis. The column chromatographic method overestimated the percentage of glycosylated hemoglobin compared to the values obtained by the electrophoretic method. This increase appeared to be proportional to the serum concentration of triglycerides. Thus, the lactescence or turbidity caused by lipid components is a matter of concern if glycosylated hemoglobin quantitation is done with ion exchange columns on whole blood samples. The problem could be magnified if the analysis is done on postprandial samples. Since hyperlipidemia is a relatively common feature of diabetes, this technical limitation of ion exchange microcolumn methods must be reckoned with. Samples with markedly elevated bilirubin may also interfere with Hb A_I quantitation in a similar fashion (20).

Sample Storage

For Hb A_I assay, blood samples are normally collected in EDTA-containing tubes. Choosing proper storage conditions for the blood samples is very critical for obtaining reproducible levels of Hb A_I with ion exchange chromatographic techniques. Prolonged storage of the blood sample even at 4°C may lead to partial oxidation of oxyhemoglobin to methemoglobin, reduction in the stability of the hemoglobin molecule, and oxidation of reduced glutathione to form oxidized glutathione, leading to the formation of Hb A_{Id} (57). The increase in Hb A_{Id} is retarded by dialysis and by sulfhydryl reagents. These changes seem to occur faster in undialyzed red cell hemolysate preparations rather than in whole blood or washed cells. Depending on the chromatographic method used, the presence of in vitro formed Hb A_{Id} may interfere with the quantitation of the true levels of Hb A_I by ion exchange chromatography. With lengthy gradi-

Table 4.3 Effect of Sample Storage on Hb A_I Values Determined by Ion Exchange Chromatography[a]

No. of days	Hb A_I (%)	
	Normal	Diabetic
0	6.3	13.7
2	6.4	13.1
7	6.2	13.0
14	5.9	12.6
22	5.9	12.8
28	6.4	12.9
35	8.6	12.9
42	8.7	14.0
50	8.8	14.5
56	10.5	15.7
Mean ± S.D.	7.4 ± 1.5	13.6 ± 1.0

[a]Samples stored as blood at 4°C.
Source: From Abraham et al. (26) by permission of the publisher.

ent elution systems in conjunction with conventional Bio-Rex 70 chromatography, Hb A_{Id} is either eluted with Hb A_o or separated from Hb A_{Ic} and Hb A_o. However, with microchromatography, Hb A_{Id} may very well be eluted with the Hb A_I fraction.

Authors differ in the reported stability of the sample at its various stages of preparation and storage. Storage of blood samples at 4°C for up to 1 month as whole blood or washed red cells did not significantly affect the Hb A_I values determined by a microcolumn procedure (10,26) (Table 4.3). In one study, a decrease in Hb A_I (10) and in another study an increase was observed after 1 month (26). Gruber and Koets (58) reported that the whole blood stored at 4°C showed significant increases in Hb A_{Ia+b} after 24 hr and in Hb A_{Ic} after 48 hr, but that stroma-free dialyzed hemolysates were stable for 7 days at 4°C and indefinitely at -140°C. Schifreen et al. (59) showed that appropriate dilution of hemolysate (50 μl of hemolysate into 3 ml of sample diluent) and addition of cysteine (25 mmol/liter) rendered both Hb A_{Ia+b} and Hb A_{Ic} stable over 5 weeks. Storage of hemolysates in glucose-free solutions for 2-3 days at

4°C may be advantageous since the contribution by the aldimine could be eliminated in this manner.

II. HIGH-PRESSURE LIQUID CHROMATOGRAPHIC SEPARATION OF GLYCOSYLATED HEMOGLOBINS

A. Bio-Rex 70 HPLC Technique

The HPLC technique described by Davis et al. (60) and by Cole et al. (61) have only minor differences in the hardware used. According to the latter group, a 0.9 X 25 cm siliconized glass analytical column (Altex, Berkeley, Calif.) is used to pack Bio-Rex 70 in high phosphate buffer (0.196 M Na^+, 0.45 M $PO_4{}^{2-}$, pH 6.42). A 50% slurry of Bio-Rex 70 is pumped into the column at a rate of 160 ml/hr until the column is filled with packed resin and pumping pressure reached 400 psi. The completed column is 9 mm X 5.8 cm. The equilibration is continued by pumping the high phosphate buffer at a rate of 23 ml/hr for 30 min. Before application of the sample, final equilibration is done with Developer 6A (0.083 M Na^+, 0.069 $PO_4{}^{2-}$, 0.016 M KCN, pH 6.82) for 30 min. After pouring the slurry into the column, the plunger is pushed down immediately without delay, until the excess buffer is removed.

The system contains basically the units acquired from different sources. Developer 6A or the high phosphate buffer flows through a bubble trap filter and a three-way slide valve to a pump, which supplies the buffer to the column. Between the pump and the column is the 7000 psi injector valve with 10-μl sample loop. The effluent from the column carrying the proteins goes through a 20-μl analytical flow cell with a dual wavelength detector. A computing integrator and a chart recorder are also connected in series to the detection device. The minor hemoglobin components are read at 405 nm at a full scale sensitivity of 0.01 optical density (OD) units, while Hb A_o is read at 546 nm at a full scale optical density of 0.08 OD. This method is adaptable to micro-use and for fast assay of Hb A_I. For fast separation of Hb A_I, a shorter (9 mm X 2.8 cm) column packed at a lower pressure (50 psi) is used. Acceptable coefficients of variation have been reported for Hb A_{Ic}, Hb A_{Ia+b}, and total Hb A_I. Standards made of Hb A_{Ic} and Hb A_o gave expected values of Hb A_{Ic} by this HPLC method.

Addition of ethanol (50 ml/liter) to the phosphate developer increases the precision by stabilizing peak shape and column activity (59). Lengthy equilibration of the column between samples is not necessary because the pK_a of the cation exchange resin is decreased from 6.10 in aqueous media to 5.9

in ethanol-water at 25°C. There is no evidence of hemoglobin denaturation due to the presence of ethanol in the developers. At the pH of the ethanolic weak and strong eluting buffers, the resin ionization is 94 and 86%, respectively. The resin ionizations are greater and more constant than in the pure aqueous system. Choosing an optimum of 200-400 mesh Bio-Rex 70 resin at low temperatures approaching 0°C may prolong the lifetime of the columns without any significant rise in the operating pressure. Low temperatures provide satisfactory separation only with a coarse resin, which would otherwise give poor performance at elevated column temperatures. Lowering the temperature increases the retention time for Hb A_{Ic}. The theoretical plate numbers also increase as the temperature reaches 0°C. Although peak width increases at lower temperatures, longer retention times offset this negative effect.

This HPLC method for quantitation of Hb A_{Ia+b} and Hb A_{Ic} has been automated by some laboratories (58,62). In one automated HPLC system, a 5-μl sample of hemolysate (240 μg of hemoglobin) is injected and chromatographed on the cation exchange resin packed to a height of 11 cm at 22°C (56). Hb A_{Ia+b} and Hb A_{Ic} are eluted sequentially within 6.4 min with the cyanide-phosphate buffer, at a constant flow rate of 3.0 ml/min. A solenoid valve activated by a programmable time-event sequence of the computing integrator makes the appropriate buffer changes at 4.2 and 15.6 min. The retention times for Hb A_{Ia+b}, Hb A_{Ic}, and Hb A_o are 0.9, 2.3, and 9.7 min, respectively. Total chromatographic time is 22 min. In another automated technique, it is possible to automate injection of up to 64 samples with the option of one to three injections per sample vial (60). The pump and chart recorder can be operated from the sample injector.

It should be pointed out that despite the claim of obtaining good resolution of Hb A_{Ia+b} and Hb A_{Ic} by these HPLC methods, the separation of Hb A_{Ia+b} from Hb A_{Ic} seems rather incomplete. However, undoubtedly, the speed of separation is considerably enhanced.

B. HPLC on Synchropak CM 300 Column

Synchropak CM 300 (Synchrom, Inc., Linden, Ind.) is a commercially available HPLC column. The cation exchanger, Synchropak CM 300, is a 6.5-μm support with a 300-Å pore diameter and a bonded polymeric coating with the functional carboxylic acid groups. Like Bio-Rex 70, this resin remains to be a mildly acidic resin, but is more suitable for operation under increased column pressure. Moreover, the resolution also should be much improved since,

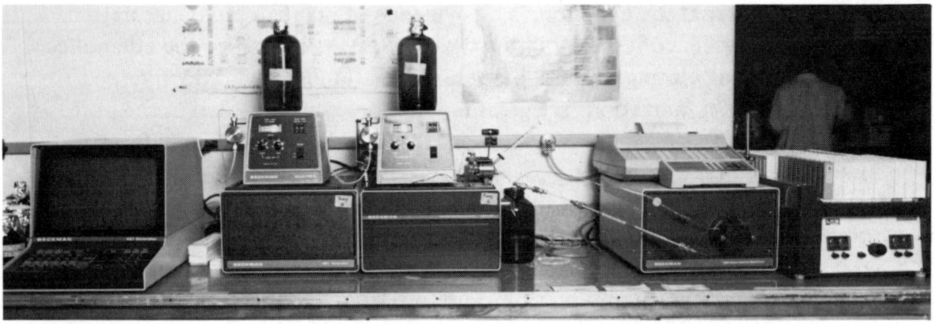

Figure 4.14 Beckman Model 330 HPLC system including Model 421 microprocessor-controller, Model 110A pumps, and Model 160 detector. A Hewlett-Packard Model 3390A recorder-integrator is also used with this system.

compared to a HPLC column packed with Bio-Rex 70 resin, this newer resin has a large number of theoretical plates. A guard column filled with Synchropak CSC packing material (Synchrom Inc., Linden, Ind.) is used with a 250 × 4.1 mm ID Synchropak CM 300 column. The basic equipment needed for a gradient elution device are two high performance HPLC pumps, gradient mixer, variable or fixed wavelength ultraviolet-visible spectrum detector, microprocessor-controller, and a recorder-integrator. Alternatively, an isocratic single-pump system without a microprocessor-controller can be used for achieving the separation of the hemoglobins if the gradient is developed externally rather than internally. The methodology described here (32,63) has been used with a Beckman Model 330 HPLC system, including Model 110A pumps, Model 160 detector, Model 421 microprocessor-controller, and a Hewlett-Packard Model 3390A recorder-integrator (Fig. 4.14).

The two developers used have the following composition: Developer A: 0.03 moles/liter Bis-Tris, 0.0015 moles/liter potassium cyanide, pH adjusted to 6.4 with acetic acid; Developer B: 0.03 moles/liter Bis-Tris, 0.15 moles/liter sodium acetate, 0.0015 moles/liter potassium cyanide, pH adjusted to 6.4 with acetic acid. Routinely, hemolysate equivalent to 300 μg of hemoglobin (5 to 10 μl freshly prepared hemolysate diluted to 25 μl with Developer A or 2- to 3-day-old hemolysates dialyzed against Developer A) are applied to the solumn and developed with a flow rate of 1 ml/min at room temperature, wavelength 405 nm (405 nm filter), 0.02 absorbance units full scale (AUFS) and 0.1 cm/min chart speed.

For separation of the glycosylated minor hemoglobin components in diabetics and in nondiabetics with or without hemoglobinopathies with a single-pump isocratic system, an externally developed sodium acetate gradient is applied. Two glass cylinders (200-ml capacity) contain either a mixture of 10% B + 90% A (cylinder A) or 75% B + 25% A (cylinder B). The column is equilibrated with the buffer in cylinder A for 20 min. For separation of the various glycosylated components, Hb A_{Ia1}, Hb A_{Ia2}, Hb A_{Ib}, Hb A_{Ic}, and Hb $A_{Id1(s)}$ (see Fig. 3.3), in adults, the column is developed isocratically with the buffer in cylinder A for the first 60 min, after which an externally developed linear gradient of sodium acetate is applied. The quality of the separation of the minor hemoglobins and their proportions are comparable to that generally seen with the lengthy Bio-Rex 70 chromatography (5). If faster separation of the glycosylated components Hb A_{Ia+b} and Hb A_{Ic} is needed, a linear gradient of sodium acetate can be supplied from the beginning of the chromatogram. For separation of the minor and the major hemoglobin components of Hb S and Hb C, a similar linear gradient of sodium acetate is applied from the beginning. The HPLC separation of the various hemoglobin components in blood samples from Hb S and Hb C homozygotes and heterozygotes are also discussed in an earlier chapter (see Chap. 3, Figs. 3.19, 3.20, 3.27, and 3.29). For separation of the glycosylated and acetylated minor hemoglobins in newborn infants by this system, the pH of the Developers A and B are adjusted to 6.2 with acetic acid and the column is developed isocratically with 10% B + 90% A for the first 60 min and for another 60 min by applying a sodium acetate gradient as described above.

The availability of a complete system containing two pumps, gradient mixer, and a microprocessor-controller makes the development and the application of a sodium acetate gradient much easier, since it is internally developed, and the column equilibration, the slope of the gradient, and the purging at the end of the run are all fully controlled by the microprocessor-controller. With this, the pH 6.4 Developers A and B are used for both adult and newborn samples. For separation of the glycosylated hemoglobins in adults, either in the absence or in the presence of abnormal hemoglobins, the column is equilibrated with 10% B (10% Developer B + 90% Developer A) for 20 min and a sodium acetate gradient is applied as follows: 10% B → 75% B, set for a duration of 120 min, and the chromatogram is completed in about 80 min. Separation of Hb A_{Ia+b}, Hb A_{Ic}, Hb A_{Id}, Hb A_o, and Hb A_2 is possible in about 1 hr (Fig. 4.15). For separation of the minor hemoglobins in cord blood samples, the column is equilibrated with 4% B for 20 min and a sodium acetate gradient is applied as follows: 4% B → 8% B

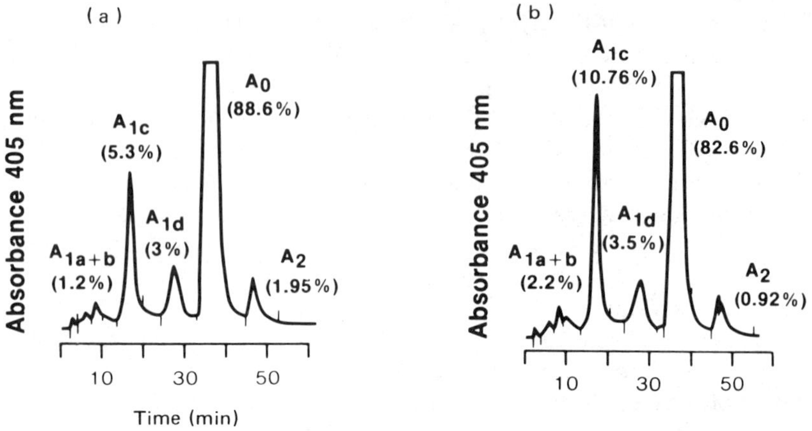

Figure 4.15 Separation of the hemoglobin components Hb A_{Ia+b}, Hb A_{Ic}, Hb A_{Id}, Hb A_o, and Hb A_2 by HPLC in a normal person (a) and a diabetic patient (b).

for 60 min and 8% B → 25% B for another 60 min. In many instances, the chromatograms are completed before 120 min. Hemoglobin Bart's, Hb F_{Ia1}, Hb F_{Ia2}, Hb F_{Ib}, and Hb F_{Ic} are readily separated in about 1 to 2 hr (see Fig. 3.12). At the end of each run the column is purged with 100% B for 10 min and reequilibrated for 20 min. Each ion exchange column is used about 100 times without significantly affecting the separation. Moreover, it should be pointed out that internally or externally developed gradients give essentially the same separation profiles for the various samples.

For separation of the aldimine Schiff base (pre-Hb A_{Ic}) from the stable Hb A_{Ic}, only a minor modification of the HPLC technique is necessary (32). The HPLC system, the column, and the developers used are essentially the same as described above. The column is equilibrated for 20 min with a mixture of 10% B and 90% A. A freshly prepared hemolysate equivalent to 200 μg of Hb is diluted to 25 μl with Developer A and immediately applied to the column. After application of the sample, the column is developed isocratically for 40 min with 10% B. Then, a gradient of 10% B → 75% B, set for a duration of 160 min, is applied. After the completion of the chromatogram in about 90 min, the column is purged with 100% B. Separation of Hb A_{Ia+b}, pre-Hb A_{Ic}, Hb A_{Ic}, Hb A_{Id}, Hb A_o, and Hb A_2 (eluted in that order) is achieved in fasting blood samples or in red cells incubated with various amounts of glucose.

Figure 4.16 demonstrates the separations of these hemoglobin components of a normal adult red cell hemolysate before and after incubation with various amounts of glucose and after treatment for aldimine elimination.

The identification of the various hemoglobin components separated by the HPLC method, except the pre-Hb A_{Ic}, was achieved by observing the chromatographic behavior on the HPLC column of individual Hb components purified by other well-established chromatographic techniques. Fifteen to 30 μg of each purified component were applied to the HPLC column and developed with the appropriate gradient system. The position on the HPLC chromatogram at which each component emerged was used to judge the identity of the various Hb components in each sample. The pre-Hb A_{Ic} was identified only by demonstrating its increase by incubation of red cells with glucose and by its disappearance under conditions that favor its removal. The pre-Hb A_{Ic} level in a fasting adult was 0.86%, and this level was increased substantially when the red cells were incubated with increasing concentrations of glucose (32) (Figs. 4.13 and 4.16). However, the pre-Hb A_{Ic} peak was absent when the incubated cells were treated with 0.05 M potassium bipthalate, pH 5.0, or when the original sample was incubated in the absence of glucose. The percentages of Hb A_{Ic} and Hb A_I determined by the HPLC method have shown good correlation with the Hb A_I values assayed by cation exchange microchromatography and glycosylated hemoglobin determined by affinity chromatography (Figs. 4.7, 4.11, 4.12, and 4.20). The percentages of the various minor and major hemoglobin components determined by HPLC and Bio-Rex 70 chromatography in 17 sickle cell anemia patients and 15 newborn infants are compared in Tables 4.4 and 4.5, respectively. When Bio-Rex 70 was used to separate the minor Hbs from SS samples, Hb F_{Ia}, Hb F_{Ib}, and Hb F_{Ic} were eluted as one peak (Hb F_I) and Hb A_2, Hb S_{Id}, and Hb S_o were eluted together. The total Hb F_I was lower for the HPLC method, but for all the other fractions the results were very similar for both the methods, with γ values ranging from 0.4 to 0.98. In the newborn samples, all the Hb components with the exception of Hb F_{Ib} and Hb A_2 gave similar values by both the methods, with γ values ranging from 0.39 to 0.8. The precision and reproducibility of the HPLC methods were also comparable to those generally seen for conventional Bio-Rex 70 methods. The obvious advantages in using HPLC are fastness, microlevel sample requirement, and rather complete and sharp separation of the several glycosylated components, including the stable and the labile Hb A_{Ic}.

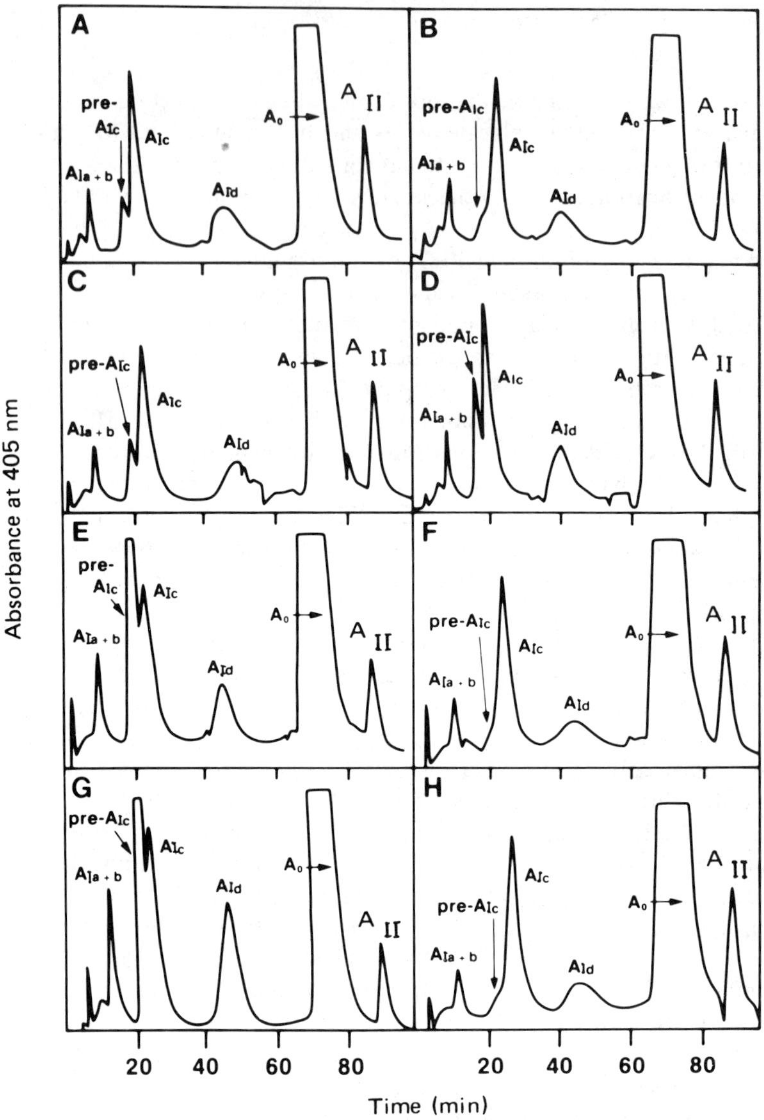

Figure 4.16 High-pressure liquid chromatographic separation of the hemoglobins in a fasting blood sample from a normal adult (A) and after incubation of the red cells at 37°C for 3 hr with the following glucose concentrations: 0 mM (B), 20 mM (C), 50 mM (D), 100 mM (E), and 200 mM (G). Chromatograms were also obtained after treatment of the incubated cells with 0.05 M potassium biphthalate, pH 5.0, for 20 min at 37°C for elimination of the aldimine. Examples are given in this figure: (F) obtained from red cells incubated with 100 mM glucose and (H) from those incubated with 200 mM glucose. From Stallings and Abraham (32).

Table 4.4 Comparison of the Levels of Various Minor Hemoglobin Components in Sickle Cell Anemia Patients as Determined by High-Pressure Liquid and Bio-Rex 70 Chromatographic Methods[a]

Method of analysis	Hb F_{Ia} (%)	Hb F_{Ib} (%)	Hb F_{Ic} (%)	Hb F_{Ia+b+c} (%)	Hb F_o (%)	Hb S_{Ia+b} (%)	Hb S_{Ic} (%)	Hb A_2 (%)	Hb S_{Id} (%)	Hb S_o (%)	Hb A_2 + Hb S_{Id} + Hb S_o (%)
HPLC	0.29±	0.52±	1.56±	2.05±	11.76±	0.18±	2.08±	2.52±	1.54±	78.45±	81.27±
	0.13	0.38	0.77	1.36	4.9	0.10	0.45	0.73	0.51	5.75	8.50
Bio-Rex 70	—	—	—	3.18±	11.59±	0.22±	2.26±	—	—	—	82.57±
	—	—	—	1.07	4.21	0.11	0.41	—	—	—	5.66
Correlation coefficient (γ)[b]	—	—	—	0.05	0.98	0.85	0.45	—	—	—	0.90

[a]Blood samples from 17 sickle cell anemia patients have been analyzed.
[b]High-pressure liquid chromatographic and Bio-Rex 70 methods are compared.
Source: From Abraham et al. (63) by permission of the C.V. Mosby Company.

Table 4.5 Comparison of the Levels of Various Minor Hemoglobin Components in Newborn Infants as Determined by High-Pressure Liquid and Bio-Rex 70 Chromatographic Methods[a]

Method of analysis	Hb Barts (%)	Hb F_{Ia1} (%)	Hb F_{Ia1} + Hb Barts (%)	Hb F_{Ia2} (%)	Hb F_{Ib} (%)	Hb F_{Ic} (%)	Hb F_o (%)	Hb A_{Id} (%)	Hb A_o (%)	Hb A_{Id} + Hb A_o (%)	Hb A_2 (%)
HPLC	0.52±	0.48±	0.91±	0.48±	1.14±	7.45±	74.37±	0.46±	15.08±	15.52±	0.16±
	0.51	0.16	0.51	0.13	0.52	0.94	4.82	0.18	5.55	5.67	0.06
Bio-Rex 70	–	–	0.85±	0.53±	2.38±	7.99±	70.44±	–	–	15.62±	2.08±
	–	–	0.65	0.15	0.31	0.62	0.62	–	–	6.65	0.93
Correlation coefficient (γ)[b]	–	–	0.81	0.85	0.14	0.45	0.85	–	–	0.87	0.27

[a]Blood samples from 15 newborn infants have been analyzed.
[b]High-pressure liquid chromatographic and Bio-Rex 70 methods are compared.
Source: From Abraham et al. (63) by permission of C. V. Mosby Company.

III. AFFINITY CHROMATOGRAPHIC QUANTITATION OF GLYCOSYLATED HEMOGLOBINS

A. Principle of the Affinity Technique

The affinity chromatographic approach is based on the fact that nonenzymatically glycosylated hemoglobin (protein) has a sugar moiety(s) attached to it. *m*-Aminophenylboronic acid immobilized on agarose or Sepharose has been used for this purpose (64-70). The primary interaction of borates or boronates with 1,2-*cis*-diol groups (Fig. 4.17) is of interest in performing biochemical separation. The borate must first be in the tetrahedral anionic form. When in this form, the borate can exchange hydroxyls with a 1,2-*cis*-diol to form a five-membered ring covalent complex. The borate-diol interaction is somewhat unusual in that although two covalent bonds are formed, the reaction is quite reversible in aqueous solution. The major structural requirements

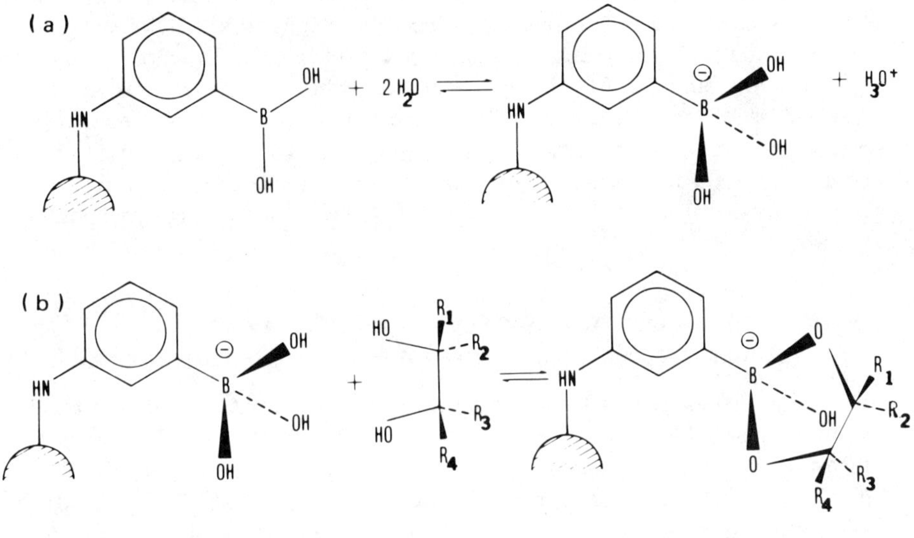

Figure 4.17 Interaction of phenyl boronate ligand with 1,2-*cis*-diol compounds. This interaction proceeds in two stages, i.e., the ionization of boronate from coplanar trigonal form to tetrahedral form (a) followed by reversible hydroxyl exchange with diol (b). From *Boronate Ligands in Biochemical Separation,* with permission granted by the publisher, Amicon Corporation.

for complex formation are that the two hydroxyls are on adjacent carbon atoms and that they are held in or can assume a coplanar configuration. In simple polyols, in which there is relatively free rotation of the hydroxyls around the carbon-carbon bonds, the strength of the interaction increases with the length of the chain. Simple diols tend to assume a trans configuration in solution and thus interact little with borate. In the case of closed ring carbohydrates, the situation is more complex because the conformation of the hydroxyls is more fixed.

In addition to polyols (primary sites), borate can interact with other sites (secondary sites) such as amines and carboxyls. In protein binding, all the primary and secondary interactions of the phenyl boronate ligand become important. Proteins contain large numbers of groups that are able to undergo hydrophobic, ionic, hydrogen-bond, and charge-transfer interactions. The pH, molarity, and divalent cations such as Mg^{2+} are important in achieving the goal of maximizing the primary boronate-diol interactions so that complete separation of glycoproteins from nonglycoproteins can be achieved. Some common buffers, such as glycine, morpholine, or HEPES (*N*-2-hydroxyethylpiperazine-*N*-2-ethanesulfonic acid), or additives, such as piperidine and ammonium salts, may promote binding. At pH below neutrality, where the boronate is unchanged, secondary interactions will become prominent. High ionic strength can be used to stamp out ionic binding or repulsion. Often pH and ionic strength operate synergistically and must be considered together. At low concentrations, Mg^{2+} reduce ionic effects effectively without causing hydrophobic binding.

B. Phenylboronate-Agarose (Sepharose) Affinity Chromatographic Quantitation of Glycosylated Hemoglobin

Phenylboronate-agarose (Sepharose) affinity gel or columns packed with this material is available from a few companies. Matrex Gel PBA-10, PBA-30, and PBA-60, were originally marketed by Amicon Corp. (Lexington, Mass.). These gels have different levels of boronate content (PBA-10 < PBA-30 < PBA-60) and are used for specific purposes (see Amicon publication *Boronate Ligands in Biochemical Separations*). Matrex Gel PBA-60 is designed for maximal binding capacity of small molecules, whereas Matrex Gel PBA-30 is designed for maximal binding of macromolecules. Matrex Gel PBA-10 is designed for macromolecular application where secondary interactions make elution from PBA-30 difficult or impossible. Successful separation of glycosylated hemoglobin is possible with Matrex Gel PBA-30. The resin is equilibrated and the column developed initially with 50 mM HEPES/NaOH, pH 8.5, or 50 mM morpholine-HCl, pH 8.5, containing 10 mM KCN. Hemolysate is applied to a column packed with the gel and washed with one of the above eluting buffers. The void volume and washings are collected and pooled ("unbound" or nonglycosylated fraction). Absorbed hemoglobins ("bound" or glycosylated fraction) is eluted with 100 mM sorbitol used as competing ions. The percentage of the glycosylated fraction is calculated on the basis of the absorbances in the Soret region (413-415 nm).

Microcolumns prepacked with 1 ml of immobilized *m*-aminophenylboronic acid on cross-linked beaded agarose, wash buffer, and elution buffers can be obtained as a kit (Glyco-GEL Test kit) from Pierce Chemical Co. (Rockford, Ill.). The column utilized a top porous frit that automatically stops the flow when the liquid level in the column reaches it. The wash buffer, which per liter contains 250 mmol of ammonium acetate, 50 mmol of magnexium chloride, and 2 g of sodium azide, pH 8.0, is used to equilibrate the column and to elute the nonglycosylated hemoglobin. A 100 mM Tris buffer, pH 8.5, containing 200 mM sorbitol, and 0.2 g/liter of sodium azide is used to elute the remaining hemoglobins. This affinity method gave total glycohemoglobin (GHb) values that correlated well with Hb A_{Ic} levels determined by HPLC and with the values of TBA assay (68). An increase in temperature of 1°C between 18° and 27°C gave a decrease of only 0.1-0.2% in GHb. Varying the pH of the first elution buffer from 7.75 to 8.25 (pH 8.0 optimum) produced only a slight change in GHb. Rechromatography by HPLC and by isoelectric focusing analysis of the glycosylated fraction obtained by the affinity separation revealed the presence of substantial population of glycosylated hemoglobins not measured by HPLC.

Isolab Inc. (Akron, Ohio) have developed another affinity microchromatographic method utilizing *m*-aminophenylboronic acid immobilized on Sepharose (Glyc-Affin System). Microcolumns are supplied prepacked with about 0.5 ml (about 0.5 cm high) affinity gel (Fig. 4.18). The columns utilize, as in other microcolumn methods, a porous frit placed just above the gel surface so that the flow stops when the liquid level in the column reaches it. Four different buffers are also supplied by the company; these are Sample Preparation Reagent (containing asparagine, $MgCl_2$, ethylmercurithiosalic acid, and sodium azide), Column Preparation Solution (containing asparagine, $MgCl_2$, ethylmercurithiosalic acid, and sodium azide), First Fraction Elution Agent (containing asparagine, $MgCl_2$, and sodium azide), and Second Fraction Elution Agent (containing sorbitol and sodium azide). The First Fraction Elution Agent may be substituted with a "homemade" buffer containing 0.05 M

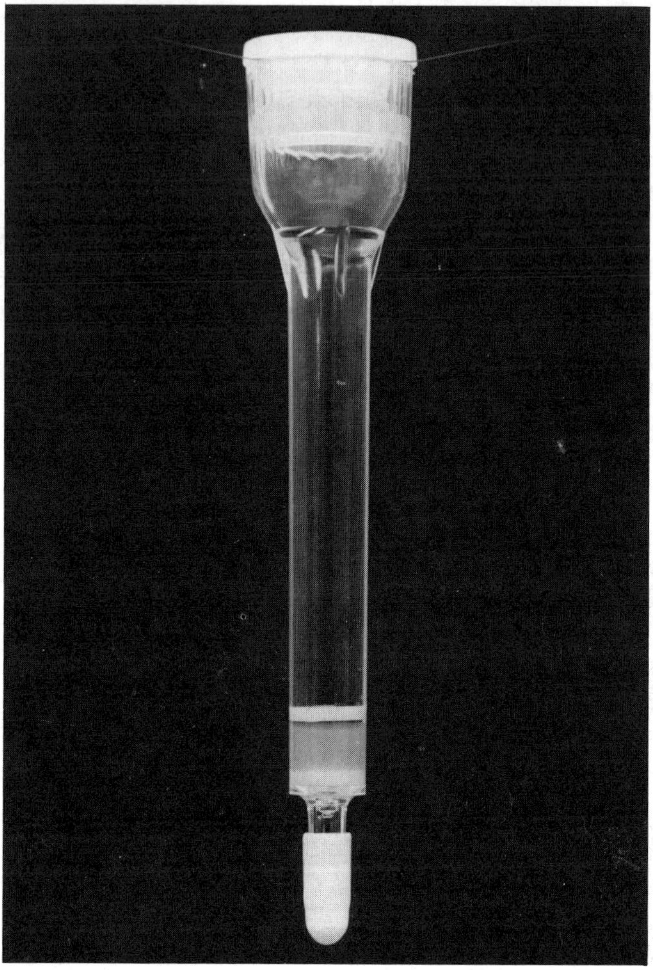

Figure 4.18 A microcolumn prepacked with *m*-aminophenylboronic acid immobilized on Sepharose (Glyc-Affin System from Isolab Inc.).

HEPES buffer, pH 8.5, containing 10 mM Mg Cl_2 and 0.02% sodium azide, and the Second Fraction Elution Agent may be substituted with 100 mM sorbital. Assay for GHb is done with saline-washed red cells or whole blood samples. Fifty microliters of the sample are mixed with 400 μl of the Sample Preparation Reagent. After equilibrating the column with 2 ml of the Column Preparation Solution, 50 μl of the hemolysate prepared as above are applied to the top of the column. The nonglycosylated hemoglobin fraction is eluted with 3 ml of the First Fraction Elution Agent. This fraction is diluted with 17 ml of deionized water. The glycohemoglobin fraction bound to the column is eluted with 2 ml of the Second Fraction Elution Agent. This fraction is not further diluted. The absorbances of the nonglycosylated (Y) and the glycosylated (X) fractions are determined at 415 nm. The percent of GHb equals 100X/(X+10Y).

The Isolab Glyc-Affin system has undergone extensive evaluation in our laboratory by performing reproducibility and correlation studies (26). Another commercially available column methodology (GLYCO-GEL Test kit, Pierce Chemical Co.) has also been subjected to similar studies (68), and the data gathered were very similar in both the systems. However, the discussion that will follow is based on the experience with the Glyc-Affin system. The precision and reproducibility of the affinity chromatographic methodology were good, with CV values within run of 1.8 and 1.1% and between run of 5.9 and 3.8% for a normal and a diabetic sample, respectively. The GHb levels determined by the affinity method correlated well with the Hb A_I levels determined by microchromatography (Fig. 4.19), Hb A_{Ic} levels determined by HPLC (Fig. 4.20), the number of glyco groups assayed fluorometrically (Fig. 4.21), and with the results of the ketoamine (TBA) assay (Fig. 4.22). The correlation coefficients were in the range of 0.91-0.97. The GHb values tended to be higher than the Hb A_I values; this was particularly noticeable in diabetic patients. This observation is explainable since the affinity gel is expected to separate the total glycosylated hemoglobins including Hb A_I and those glycosylated at sites other than the β-chain amino terminus. The mean level of Hb A_I (6.0 ± 0.8%; 4.2-7.6%) was not significantly different from the GHb level (6.3 ± 0.6%; 5.0-7.4%) in the same group of normals. In the diabetic patients, however, the mean and the ranges of GHb were significantly higher (13.0 ± 2.6%, 9.4-18.9%, for Hb A_I vs. 16.4 ± 4.0%, 9.1-24.1, for GHb).

Changes in Hb A_I levels due to ambient temperature variations and sample storage are two common problems in glycosylated hemoglobin assay with cation exchange microchromatography. It seems that affinity chromatography is not substantially influenced by these factors (26,69). Between 4° and 17°C, there was only a slight increase in GHb, but, between 17° and 35°C, no signifi-

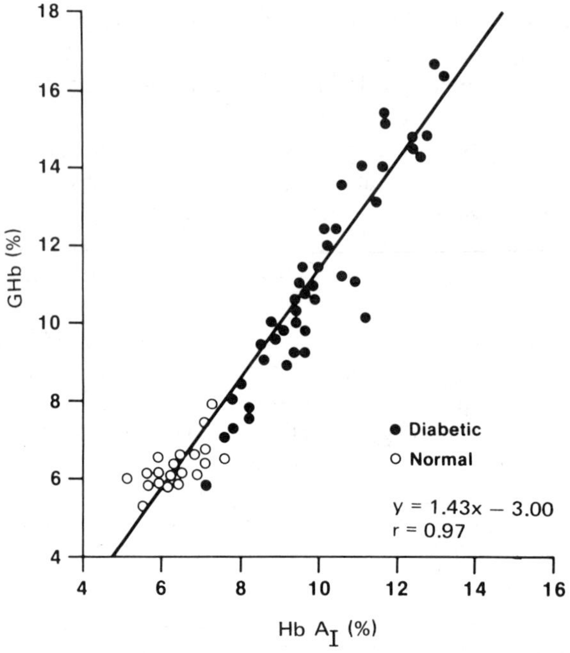

Figure 4.19 Correlation of the percentage GHb values determined by affinity chromatography (Glyc-Affin System, Isolab Inc.) with the percentage Hb A_I values determined by cation exchange microchromatography (Fast Hemoglobin Test System, Isolab Inc.) in normal controls and in diabetics. From Abraham et al. (26) with minor modifications; by permission of the C. V. Mosby Company.

cant change was observed (Table 4.6). Hb A_I, at the same time, increased drastically with increasing temperatures. Thus, for all practical reasons, affinity columns are developed at room temperature, and no correction is made for any moderate variations in temperature. Storing blood samples at 4°C for up to 2 months apparently did not affect the levels of GHb as determined by the affinity method (Table 4.6), whereas Hb A_I levels increased after 30 days of storage (26) (Table 4.3).

The labile aldimine has been shown to influence the levels of Hb A_I determined by cation exchange microchromatography to a great extent. It seems that by affinity chromatography only the ketoamine, not the aldimine, form of Hb A_I

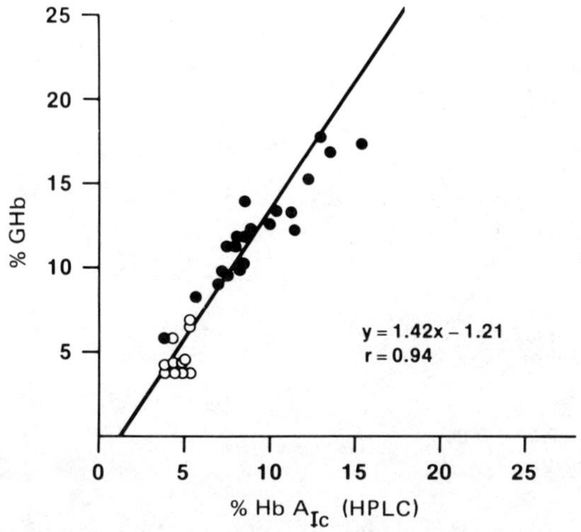

Figure 4.20 Correlation of the Hb A_{Ic} levels determined by cation exchange HPLC on Synchropak CM 300 columns with the levels of GHb in normal controls (○) and in diabetics (●).

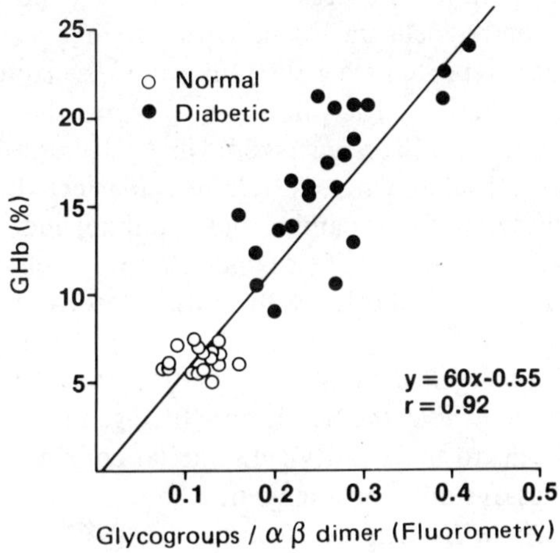

Figure 4.21 Correlation of the number of glyco groups determined fluorometrically with the GHb levels in normals and diabetics.

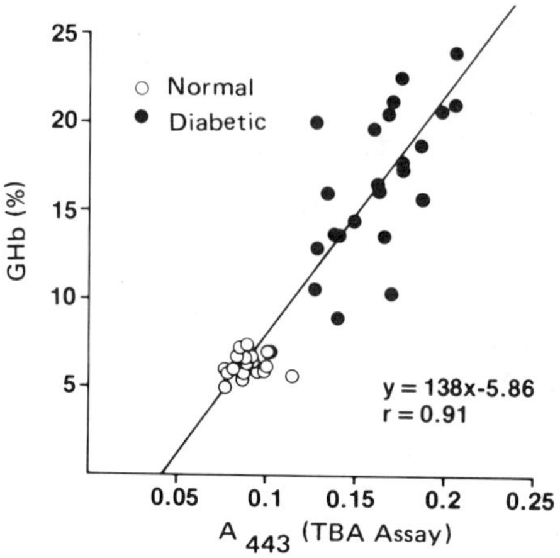

Figure 4.22 Correlation of the TBA assay values (A_{443}) and GHb levels.

is quantitated. This conclusion was made based on the data presented in Table 4.8. Two samples, a normal and a diabetic, are included in this study. The percentage of Hb A_I by the ion exchange method and the percentage of GHb by the affinity method were determined simultaneously on fasting and postprandial blood samples and also on red cells incubated with 100 mM glucose for 3 hr at 37°C. The assays were repeated after the removal of the labile aldimine by incubation of the red cells in saline for 4 hr at 37°C. When the fasting and 1½ hr postprandial blood samples were analyzed, Hb A_I decreased significantly after the removal of the aldimine, whereas GHb was unaffected. This indicated that Hb A_I value included both ketoamine and aldimine, and the GHb value seemed to include only ketoamine. This conclusion was well substantiated by assaying the glucose-incubated cells. Substantial increase in Hb A_I was noticed, while GHb remained the same. Most noteworthy was the observation that after the reduction of the Schiff base with $NaBH_4$, the GHb values increased markedly. Thus, it seems that the Schiff base linkage readily dissociates when the sugar moiety binds to the affinity gel. Similar conclusions were made on the basis of the assays done on a large number of samples before and after incubation of red cells with saline for 5 hr at 37°C (68).

The application of ion exchange chromatography, microchromatography in particular, has been limited to samples containing no Hb F and no abnormal hemoglobins. The quantitation of the GHb is possible with the affinity chro-

Table 4.6 Effect of Ambient Temperature on the Quantitation of GHb and Hb A_I by the Affinity Method

Temperature (°C)	Sample source[a]	GHb (%)	Hb A_I (%)
4	Normal	5.2	1.6
4	Diabetic	15.0	1.9
9	Normal	5.6	2.1
9	Diabetic	15.9	2.4
17	Normal	5.9	5.2
17	Diabetic	17.3	9.1
25	Normal	6.0	8.0
25	Diabetic	18.0	13.7
30	Normal	5.6	18.5
30	Diabetic	17.8	28.5
35	Normal	4.9	37.3
35	Diabetic	17.6	43.1

[a]Samples stored as blood at 4°C.
Source: From Abraham et al. (26) by permission of the publisher.

matographic approach even in the presence of Hb F and abnormal variants such as Hb S and Hb C (26,70). The GHb values should represent the total glycosylated hemoglobins, the products of glycosylation of different sites on different hemoglobins present in a hemolysate. Table 4.9 compares the GHb values with the results of the TBA assay for ketoamine and the fluorometric assay for glyco groups in newborn infants and in persons with some hemoglobinopathies. Reasonable correlations of the GHb values with the results of the chemical assays were noticed. These studies show that the presence of Hb F, Hb S, or Hb C does not interfere with the affinity method as well as with the chemical methods.

C. Identification of the Hemoglobins Separated by Affinity Chromatography

In affinity chromatography glycosylated Hb binds to the affinity gel through its sugar moiety(s) that involves *cis*-diol-boronate covalent linkage. Although

Table 4.7 Effect of Sample Storage on GHb Values Determined by Affinity Chromatography[a]

No. of days	GHb (%) Normal	GHb (%) Diabetic
0	6.6	17.7
2	7.1	18.7
7	6.8	17.9
14	6.9	16.6
22	7.3	17.0
28	6.5	17.4
35	6.4	17.8
42	6.1	18.3
50	6.4	18.5
56	6.4	18.5
Mean ± S.D.	6.6 ± 0.4	17.7 ± 0.6

[a]Samples were stored as blood at 4°C.

Source: From Abraham et al. (26) by permission of the publisher.

this binding appears to be a straightforward phenomenon, the nature of the sugar moiety and the binding sites and certain conformational constraints may influence this binding process. So, it is important to find out the hemoglobin types and their quantities in the glycosylated (bound) and the nonglycosylated (unbound) fractions. To achieve this, it was necessary to isolate affinity column fractions and rechromatograph them using Bio-Rex 70 macrocolumns (26) or subject them to HPLC (68). To isolate appreciable amounts of the glycosylated and the nonglycosylated fractions, 30 mg Hb was applied to a 1 × 10 cm macrocolumn of the phenylboronate-Sepharose affinity gel and developed with the same developers used with the microcolumn method (Fig. 23) (26). Red cell hemolysate equivalent to 30 mg Hb from a normal adult and a diabetic patient and the glycosylated and the nonglycosylated fractions isolated from a similar quantity of each hemolysate were rechromatographed on Bio-Rex 70 columns (Fig. 4.24). The glycosylated fraction contained 9.5% Hb A_{Ia+b}, 52.3% Hb A_{Ic}, and 38.1% Hb A_o-like (presumably

Table 4.8 Effect of Labile Aldimine on the Measurement of Glycosylated Hemoglobin by Affinity Chromatography and Hb A_I by Ion Exchange Chromatography

Sample source	Treatment	Hb A_I (%)	GHb (%)
Normal	Fasting	5.8	5.5
Diabetic		13.8	17.0
Normal	After aldimine removal	5.2	5.7
Diabetic		11.1	16.8
Normal	1½ hr postprandial	6.2	5.7
Diabetic		14.4	17.2
Normal	After aldimine removal	5.6	5.7
Diabetic		11.5	16.9
Normal	100 mM glucose + RBC, 3 hr	11.8	5.9
Diabetic		17.1	15.9
Normal	After reduction with NaBH	12.0	12.6
Diabetic		16.1	22.7
Normal	After aldimine removal	6.4	6.7
Diabetic		12.1	16.5

Source: From Abraham et al. (26) by permission of the publisher.

glycosylated at sites other than the β-chain amino terminus) components in the diabetic sample. The nonglycosylated hemoglobin fraction contained, in addition to Hb A_o, a small amount of Hb A_{Ic} and a large proportion of Hb A_{Ia+b}. On the basis of electrophoretic analysis, the Hb A_{Ic} peak of the nonglycosylated fraction was predominantly Hb F. About 29% of the total Hb A_{Ia+b}, 67% Hb A_{Ic}, and 7% Hb A_o (calculated on the basis of the quantities of the corresponding components in the total hemolysate taken as 100%) appeared in the glycosylated fraction. Similar conclusions could be made from the analysis of the glycosylated and the nonglycosylated fractions and the total hemolysate from the normal adult. One striking difference was noteworthy, i.e., glycosylated Hb A_o was normally only 3% of the total Hb A_o, whereas in the diabetic, it

Table 4.9 Comparison of Affinity Chromatographic, Fluorometric, and Colorimetric Methods for Quantitation of Glycosylated Hemoglobin in Newborn Infants and in Some Hemoglobinopathies[a]

Sample	Hb type	GHb (%)[b]	Glyco groups/$\alpha\beta$[c]	A_{443}[d]
Newborn (25)	FA	4.1 ± 0.7	0.067 ± 0.008	0.083 ± 0.004
HPFH homozygote (1)	FF	5.2	0.076	0.077
HPFH heterozygote with uncontrolled diabetes (1)	AF	20.0	0.328	0.147
Sickle cell trait (16)	AS	6.7 ± 0.9	0.130 ± 0.023	0.102 ± 0.009
Sickle cell anemia (20)	SS	3.9 ± 0.7	0.062 ± 0.015	0.081 ± 0.012
SC condition (1)	SC	5.3	0.056	0.069
SC condition with controlled diabetes (1)	SC	7.2	0.072	0.074

[a]Results are expressed as mean ± standard deviation.
[b]Percentage of glycosylated hemoglobin determined by affinity chromatography.
[c]The glyco groups were determined by fluorometry.
[d]The TBA assay was used for the A_{443} determination.
[e]Number of samples analyzed shown in parentheses.

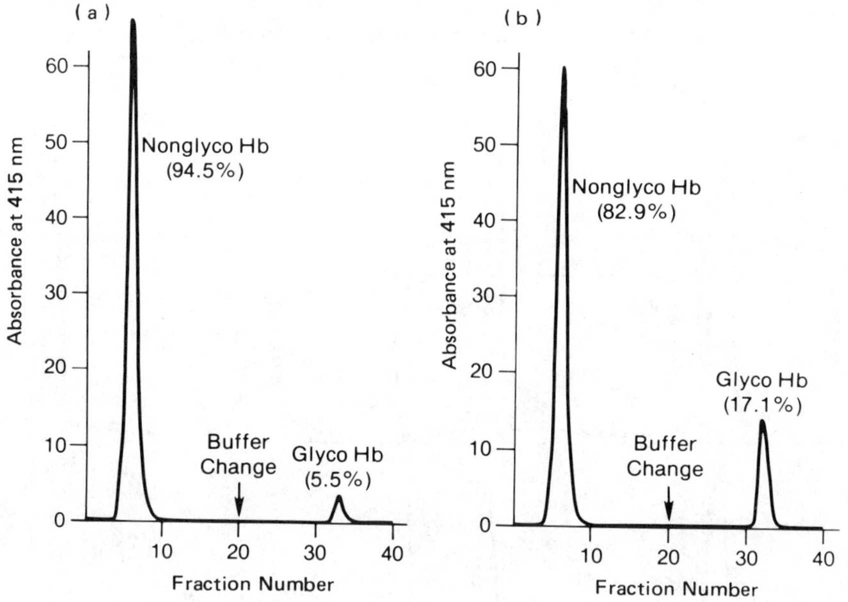

Figure 4.23 Preparative affinity chromatographic separation of glycosylated hemoglobins (glyco Hb) and nonglycosylated hemoglobins (nonglyco Hb) in red cell hemolysates of a normal adult and a diabetic patient. Thirty milligrams of Hb were applied to a column (1 × 10 cm) of phenylboronate-Sepharose and developed first with the First Fraction Elution Agent and then with the Second Fraction Elution Buffer (buffer change), and fractions of 1.5 ml were collected. From Abraham et al. (26) by permission of the C. V. Mosby Company.

Table 4.10 Chemical Analysis (TBA Assay) of Isolated Hb Components from Glycosylated and Nonglycosylated Fractions

Affinity gel fractions	Bio-Rex 70 fractions	TBA (A_{443})
Glycosylated	A_{Ia+b}	0.348
	A_{Ic}	0.560
	A_o	0.140
Nonglycosylated	A_{Ia+b}	0.099
	A_{Ic}	0.062
	A_o	0.046
Total (unfractionated)	A_{Ia+b}	0.204
	A_{Ic}	0.386
	A_o	0.056

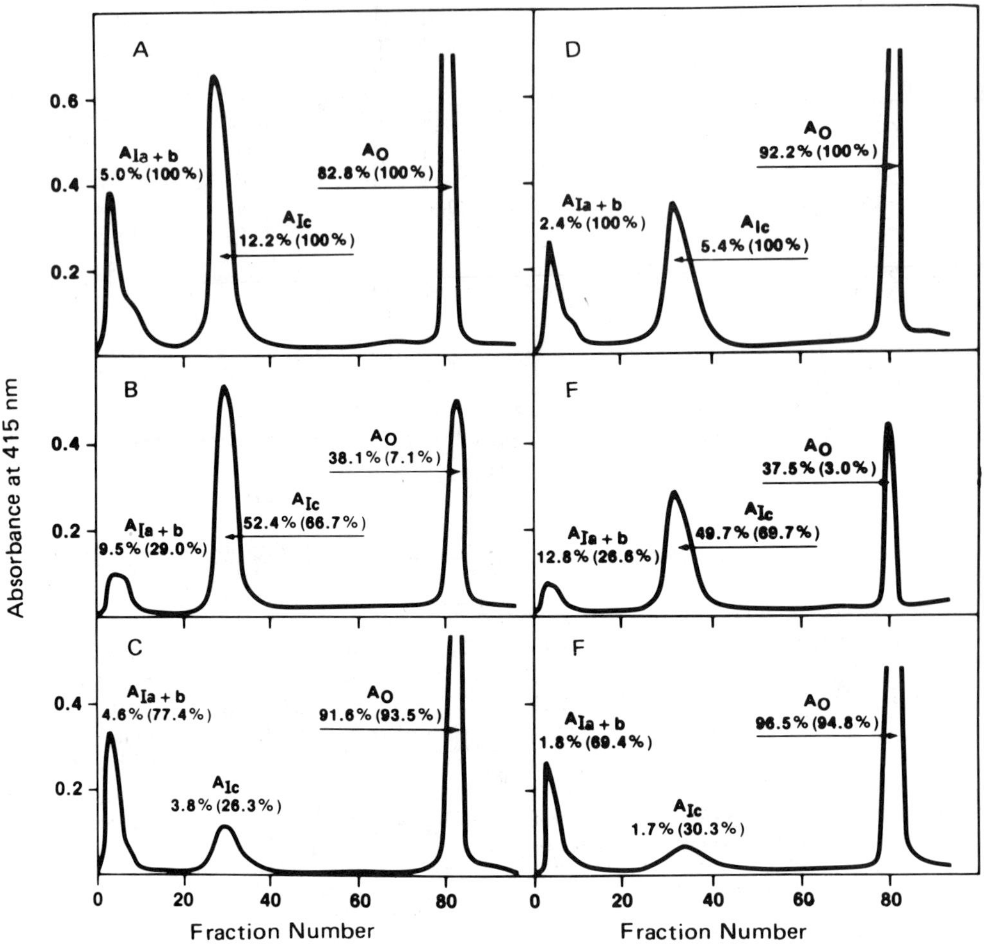

Figure 4.24 Rechromatography on Bio-Rex 70 columns of glycosylated (glyco) and nonglycosylated (nonglyco) fractions isolated by affinity chromatography. These fractions and the unfractionated hemolysates from a diabetic patient (A-C) and a normal adult (D-F) were chromatographed on Bio-Rex 70 columns according to the classical Trivelli method. The percentages given in parentheses represent the recoveries and were calculated by taking the quantities of the corresponding component in the total hemolysate as 100%. The other percentages represent the distribution of each component within a given fraction. From Abraham et al. (26) by permission of the C. V. Mosby Company.

was about 7%. Thus, Hb A_{Ic} and glycosylated Hb A_o were significantly elevated in the diabetic patient. The thiobarbituric acid assay of the total sample and the glycosylated and the nonglycosylated fractions, as expected, showed considerable enrichment of ketoamine in the glycosylated fraction and very little in the nonglycosylated fraction (Table 4.10). Hemoglobin A_{Ia+b}, Hb A_{Ic}, and Hb A_o components isolated from the glycosylated fraction contained significant amounts of ketoamine. The ketoamine content of glycosylated Hb A_o was apparently low, probably because 5-HMF was not readily released from the glycosylated lysines. The corresponding components from the nonglycosylated fractions have significantly lower levels of ketoamine. It is surprising that about 70% of the total Hb A_{Ia+b} was eluted as a part of the nonglycosylated fraction. This apparently is not due to an inefficiency of the glycosylated hemoglobins in the Hb A_{Ia+b} to bind to the affinity gel. This is supported by the observation that the Hb A_{Ia+b} of the nonglycosylated fraction contains significantly lower amounts of ketoamine. Thus, it appears that, by conventional Bio-Rex 70 chromatographic approach, the true levels of Hb A_{Ia+b} is overestimated, since some other modified hemoglobin(s) seem to cochromatograph with the true glycosylated Hb A_{Ia+b}.

Only 11.8% of the total Hb F_{Ia+b} that is originally present in a cord blood hemolysate and 6.8% of Hb F_{Ic}, 1.2% of Hb F_o, and 1.7% Hb A_o appeared in the glycosylated fraction (69) (Fig. 4.25). The percentage distribution of Hb F_{Ia+b}, Hb F_{Ic}, Hb F_o, and Hb A_o in the glycosylated fraction was 10.8, 9.0, 59.9, and 11.1%, respectively. It is not totally unexpected to find that only a small portion of Hb F_{Ic} is eluted with the glycosylated fraction, because Hb F_{Ic} is mostly an acetylated component although a glycosylated component (glucose adduct) may cochromatograph with this Hb component. As with Hb A_{Ia+b} in adult samples, only a small fraction of Hb F_{Ia+b} is eluted with the glycosylated hemoglobin from an affinity column. Either Hb F_{Ia+b} is poorly retained by the affinity gel or a majority of the hemoglobins in this minor component is not in the glycosylated form. The results of chemical analysis of the hemoglobin fractions in the glycosylated and nonglycosylated fractions strongly support the latter possibility. It is indeed quite surprising to see that about 60% of the glycosylated hemoglobin in a cord blood sample is Hb F_o-like, which is presumably formed by glycosylation of the α-chain amino terminus and the ϵ-NH_2 groups of lysyl residues on both the α and the γ chains. It seems that these sites are preferred over the γ-chain NH_2 terminus in the glycosylation of Hb F_o.

It should be interesting to see what effect the heterozygosity or homozygosity for an abnormal hemoglobin would have on the distribution of the various glycosylated minor hemoglobins in the glycosylated fraction isolated by affinity chromatography. The glycosylated and the nonglycosylated

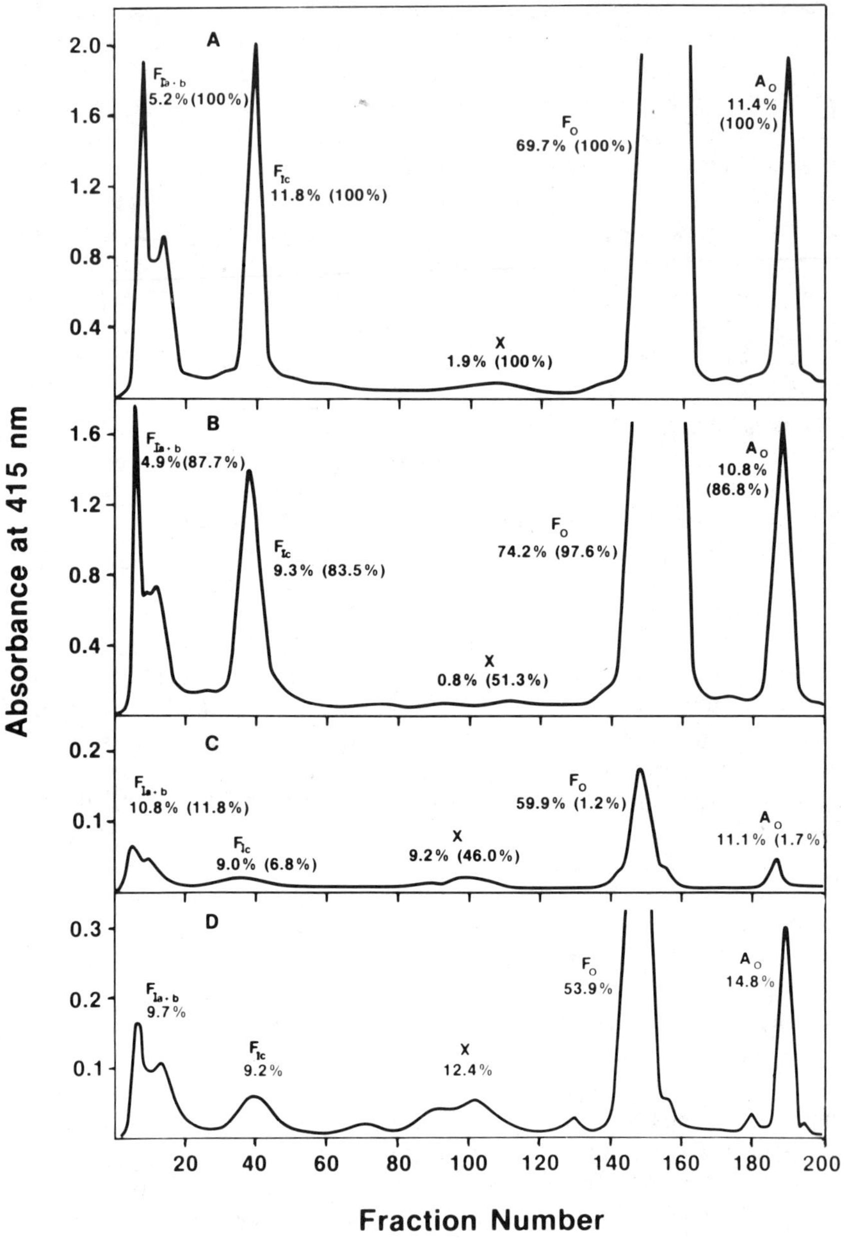
Absorbance at 415 nm
A
F_{Ia+b} 5.2% (100%)
F_{Ic} 11.8% (100%)
X 1.9% (100%)
F_O 69.7% (100%)
A_O 11.4% (100%)
B
F_{Ia+b} 4.9% (87.7%)
F_{Ic} 9.3% (83.5%)
X 0.8% (51.3%)
F_O 74.2% (97.6%)
A_O 10.8% (86.8%)
C
F_{Ia+b} 10.8% (11.8%)
F_{Ic} 9.0% (6.8%)
X 9.2% (46.0%)
F_O 59.9% (1.2%)
A_O 11.1% (1.7%)
D
F_{Ia+b} 9.7%
F_{Ic} 9.2%
X 12.4%
F_O 53.9%
A_O 14.8%
Fraction Number

Hb fractions isolated by affinity chromatography from a sickle cell heterozygote and from a homozygote were also analyzed by both Bio-Rex 70 chromatography and HPLC (M. Stallings et al., unpublished information). The glycosylated hemoglobin fraction from a sickle cell heterozygote contained 10.1, 23.0, 5.4, 15.3, 21.4, and 15.1% Hb A_{Ia+b}, Hb A_{Ic}, Hb S_{Ia+b}, Hb S_{Ic}, glycosylated Hb A_o, and glycosylated Hb S_o, respectively. The glycosylated hemoglobin isolated from a sickle cell anemia patient contained, in addition to Hb F_I, Hb F_o, and Hb A_2, about 2% Hb S_{Ia+b}, 30% Hb S_{Ic}, and 39% Hb S_o. The results showed a substantial enrichment of the Hb S_{Ia+b} and Hb S_{Ic} components in the glycosylated fraction as compared to the total hemolysate.

IV. AGAR GEL ELECTROPHORESIS

A complete separation of Hb A_I from Hb A_o has not been possible by electrophoresis at alkaline pH either by starch gel electrophoresis or by electrophoresis on cellulose acetate plates, which are most commonly used for hemoglobin electrophoresis for the purpose of primary screening for abnormal hemoglobins. Agar gel electrophoresis seems to be the method of choice for electrophoretic separation of Hb A_I. However, the separation of the constituent components of Hb A_I is not possible by this approach.

Allen et al. (71) described a system for separating and quantitating Hb A_I by agar gel electrophoresis and gel scanning. This method was modified by other investigators and compared with reference HPLC and chemical methods (72,73). The essential features of the methodology are described here: Prepare a mixture, per liter, of 20 g agar (Difco, Detroit, Mich.), 40 g sorbitol, 35 mmol sodium citrate, 25 mmol citric acid, 0.9 mmol disodium EDTA; if necessary, adjust pH to 6.3. Heat this mixture until the compo-

---

Figure 4.25 Rechromatography on Bio-Rex 70 columns of the glycosylated (glyco) and the nonglycosylated (nonglyco) fractions isolated by affinity chromatography from red cell hemolysate of a newborn infant. The glyco (C) and the nonglyco (B) fractions isolated from 200 mg red cell hemolysate and the unfractionated and equally treated total hemolysate (A) were applied to 2 X 30 cm Bio-Rex 70 columns and developed with a sodium phosphate gradient. (D) shows the separation of the Hbs in 23 mg of the glyco fraction isolated from 500 mg hemolysate. The percentages given in parenthesis represent the recoveries and were calculated taking the quantities of the corresponding component in the total hemolysate as 100%. The other percentages give the distribution of each component within a given fraction. From Abraham et al. (69).

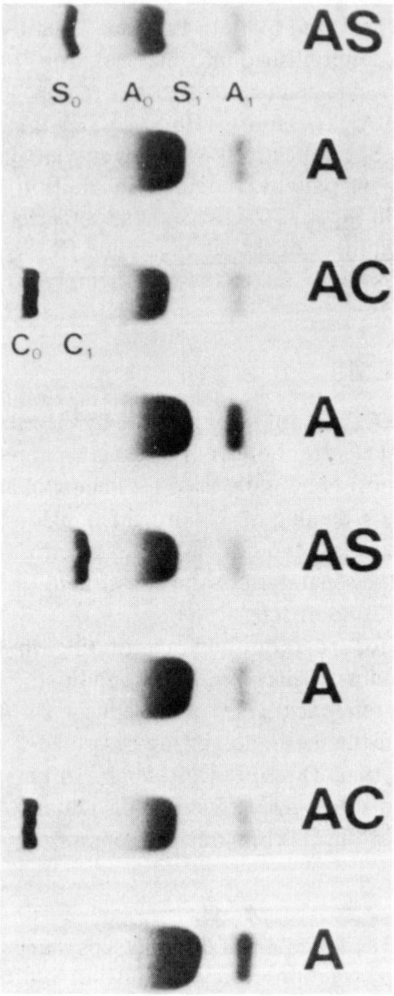

Figure 4.26 Agar gel electrophoretic pattern of hemoglobin components in normals, Hb S traits, and Hb C traits. At the end of the electrophoresis the gel was stained with Amido Black 10 B solution. Anode to the left. Courtesy of Aleyassine et al. (73) by permission of the editor of *Clinical Chemistry*.

nents are dissolved completely, and the gel is cast on a flexible polyester film (Corning Medical and Scientific, Medfield, Mass.). Hemolysate is prepared by mixing one part of whole blood with three prts of a hemolyzing agent containing saponin. All the necessary electrophoretic equipment are commercially available (Corning Medical and Scientific). Place 1 μl of hemolysate into each of eight wells in the agar gel. Add glycosylated hemoglobin buffer (95 ml) to each electrode chamber. Insert the agar gel into the casette holder of the electrophoresis cell cover, agar side facing out. Apply 60 V for 40 min, then place the gel in a 55°C oven for 120 min. The minor components (Hb A_I, Hb S_I, Hb C_I) are well separated from their respective major Hb components (Fig. 4.26). The proportion of Hb components are determined by scanning densitometry (Figs. 4.27 and 4.28). It seems that the voltage (60 V) and time (40 min) are very critical for obtaining optimum separations. It may be necessary to screen different batches of agar material and choose the one that provides the best separation.

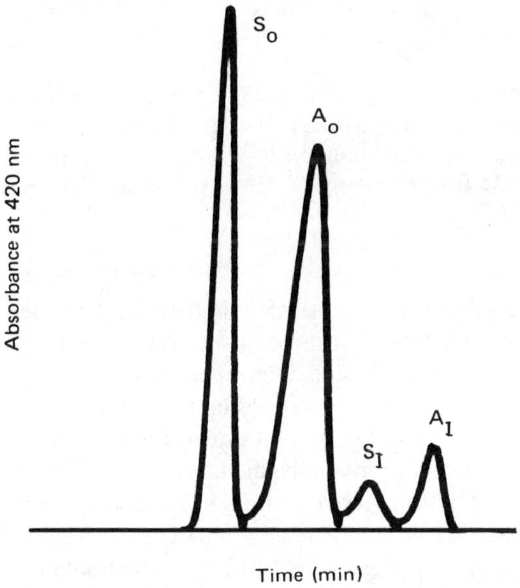

Figure 4.27 Electrophoretic distribution of the minor and the major hemoglobin components in a blood sample from a Hb S heterozygote who was also diabetic, as recorded by scanning densitometry at 420 nm after agar gel electrophoresis. Hb A_I = 8.5%; Hb S_I = 6.6%; Hb A_o = 48.8%; Hb S_o = 36.1%. Courtesy of Aleyassine et al. (73) by permission of the editor of *Clinical Chemistry*.

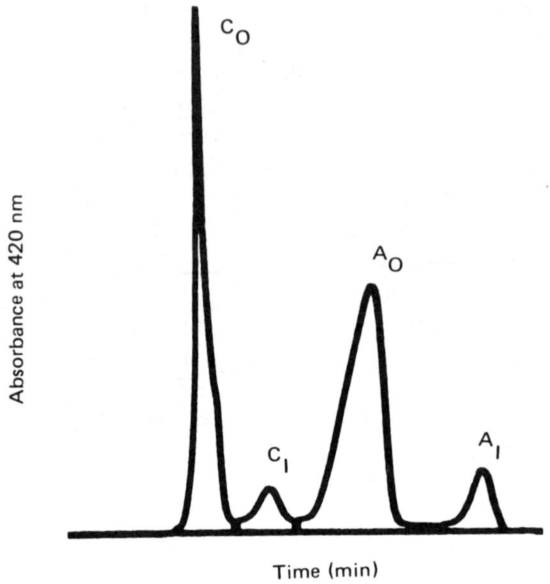

Figure 4.28 Electrophoretic distribution of hemoglobin component in a blood sample from a Hb C heterozygote who was also diabetic, as recorded by scanning densitometry at 420 nm after agar gel electrophoresis. Hb A_I = 8.2%; Hb A_o = 51.4%; Hb C_I = 5.4%; Hb C_o = 35.0%. Courtesy of Aleyassine et al. (73) by permission of the editor of *Clinical Chemistry*.

The precision and reproducibility (CV) of this method are in the generally acceptable range, despite being higher than those of the column methods. In contrast to ion exchange column methods, the determination of Hb A_I by agar gel electrophoresis is insensitive to minor variations in pH, ionic strength, and temperature. Even at the extremes of 19° or 37°C, quantitation is unaffected. Moreover, unlike the ion exchange methods, quantitation of glycosylated hemoglobin is not affected by the presence of abnormal hemoglobin variants S or C. In fact, Hb S_I and Hb C_I can be readily separated and quantitated by this electrophoretic approach (Figs. 4.26-4.28) (73). It should be pointed out, however, that none of these hemoglobin components have been properly identified. The quantitative differences in these minor hemoglobins in nondiabetics and in diabetics before and after undergoing treatment has been used as evidence to identify them as glycosylated hemoglobins. As with ion exchange column methods, Hb F can interfere with Hb A_I quantitation. With three electrophoretic cells and a power supply, 24 samples can be completed in

75 min. This electrophoretic method appears to be suited for routine use in clinical laboratory for quantitation of total Hb A_I.

V. ISOELECTRIC FOCUSING

Isoelectric focusing (IEF) offers a more definitive and precise means of separating hemoglobins or proteins in general. It is an alternative method for separating proteins on the basis of their surface charge and, under proper conditions, can resolve proteins whose isoelectric points differ as little as 0.02 pH unit. The potential of this technique in separating hemoglobins was demonstrated by Svensson (74), who introduced shallow pH gradients by electrolysis of carrier ampholytes in sucrose density gradients. Nevertheless, better resolution can be obtained by developing the pH gradient in a medium such as polyacrylamide that restricts diffusion and stabilizes the protein bands. The separation of hemoglobins by isoelectric focusing in polyacrylamide gels was described by Drysdale et al. in 1971 (75). Since the pIs of most of the human hemoglobins lie between pH 6.7 and 7.7 (probably with the exception of some acidic minor Hbs), ampholytes with a pH range of 6-8 are well suited for this purpose. In this isoelectric focusing technique, the gel contains 4% and 2% (w/v) acrylamide and ampholyte (pH 6-8), respectively. Gel polymerization is done in tubes (10 × 0.3 cm inner diameter) that are sealed at one end with dialysis membrane. Polymerization is initiated by the addition of 0.02% (w/v) of both *N,N,N′N′*-tetramethylethylenediamine (TEMED) and ammonium persulfate. Gel electrofocusing is conducted in an apparatus similar to those commonly used for "disc" electrophoresis. The tubes are contained between the electrolyte vessels in a jacket through which cold water is circulated. Solution (50 ml) of 0.02 M phosphoric acid (pH 2.2) and 0.01 M NaOH (pH 12.0) are used as anolyte and catholyte, respectively. Only the tips of the tubes are in contact with the electrolytes. Platinum electrodes are arranged close to the extremities of the tubes to minimize pH and concentration gradients. To eliminate excess persulfate, the gels are prerun for 10 min with a current of 1 mA/tube. About 200 μg of hemoglobin in a volume of 10-30 μl are applied on top of the gel in a solution of ampholyte (4%, w/v). The current is restored to 1 mA/tube until the voltage reaches 500 V; the voltage is then maintained at this level throughout. At the end of the run, the gels are scanned at 576 nm. The pH gradient can be assessed by sectioning the gels, eluting the gels into water, and by determining the pH of the eluate. A variety of normal and abnormal hemoglobin variants can be separated by this approach. Hemoglobin A_I isolated by column chromatography gives four bands, namely, Hb F_o, Hb A_{Ic}, Hb A_{Ib}, and Hb A_{Ia} separated in that order. However, the separation of Hb A_{Ic} from Hb A_o in whole hemolysate is incomplete, and, thus, direct quantitation of total Hb A_I is not possible with this approach. Better separation is possible by fractionating the ampholyte preparation to form more shallow pH gradients. In fact, several laboratories have improved this technique so that quantitation of Hb A_{Ic} is readily possible.

Thin-layer isoelectric focusing technique may be successfully applied to separate various hemoglobin variants and minor components. The procedure, as described by Basset et al. (76) for preparation of a gel of 250 × 115 × 0.5 mm, is as follows: A stock solution of acrylamide contains 9.7 g acrylamide, 0.3 g bisacrylamide, and 50 ml of distilled water. To 4.5 ml of this solution, 0.9 ml of 40% ampholines (pH 6-8), 0.9 ml of 40% ampholines (pH 7-9), and 11.7 ml of distilled water are added. After degassing, 3.5 μl of TEMED and finally a 3% ammonium persulfate solution (0.18 ml) are added. The final mixture is poured immediately between the plates. Polymerization occurs within a few minutes. After standing for 1 hr, the gel between the two plates is placed for 1 hr in a humidified chamger at 4°C. Focusing is done at 10°C with the LKB Multiphor apparatus using a constant power of 18 W. Utilization of a mixture of equal quantities of ampholines of pH 6.0-8.0 and pH 7.0-9.0 allows good resolution of bands along the entire length of the gradient. Up to 48 samples can be applied on a single plate. Hemoglobin A_{Ic}, Hb F_o, and Hb A_o can be separated from each other. Also, a large number of hemoglobin variants can be separated by this method. With a similar isoelectric focusing system utilizing high-resolution microdensitometry, blood samples from normals and diabetics were analyzed for Hb A_{Ic}, and the results showed an excellent correlation with the glycosylated Hb levels determined by the conventional Bio-Rex 70 method (77). In addition, finger stick samples were found to give equivalent results to venipuncture samples. A modified type of IEF consists of transforming a linear pH gradient into a nonlinear one by the addition of an amphoteric substance with an isoelectric point close to the pIs of the two hemoglobins (78). The dipeptide histidylglycine is very efficient in flattening the pH gradient in the hemoglobin region. Even when added at low concentrations (10-100 mM), full resolution of Hb A_{Ic} and Hb A_o is achieved.

Mortensen (79,80) used ampholine polyacrylamide gel (PAG) plate, pH 5-6.5 (LKB-Produkter AB, Bromma, Sweden) to separate glycosylated hemoglobins. The introduction of a more acidic, narrow pH range of ampholytes has enabled to differentiate Hb A_o, Hb A_{Ic}, and the pre-A_{Ic}. Pre-A_{Ic} will be focused anodal to Hb A_{Ic}. The proportion of each Hb component is determined by cutting out the bands and extracting with 0.05 M ammonium bicarbonate. The extracts are measured spectrophotometrically. Alternanatively, the hemoglobin bands may be scanned after staining. Similar separation of the two types of Hb A_{Ic} was also achieved by Welinder and Svendsen (81) without choosing ampholytes with a narrow or acidic pH range. The gels are made of 5% Cyanogum 41 (95% acrylamide, 5% bisacrylamide), 2% ampholine, pH 7-9; 0.1% ampholine, pH 3.5-10; 2% β-alanine; and 0.02% riboflavine (all w/v). Gels of 1 mm thickness are photopolymerized for 1-2 hr and prefocused for 1 hr at 500 V.

Despite the fact that IEF requires specialized equipments and uses rather expensive ampholines, it is an attractive alternate to ion exchange column methods because it gives satisfactory separation of Hb A_{Ic} from Hb F. Samples with very high levels of Hb F, however, can potentially interfere with the quantitation of Hb A_{Ic} because Hb F_I may comigrate with Hb A_{Ic}. The IEF also seems to have the great potential of separating the glycosylated components of abnormal variants. It is surprising that even under conditions that are favorable for the separation of pre-Hb A_{Ic} from Hb A_{Ic}, the other minor Hbs A_{Ia1}, A_{Ia2}, or A_{Ib}, are not separated in detectable amounts from red cell hemolysates (79). However, separation of Hb A_{Ia} and Hb A_{Ib} are possible with isolated Hb A_I (75).

VI. IMMUNOASSAY

Radioimmunoassays are available that are capable of recognizing and, if necessary, quantifying hemoglobin variants S, C, D, and E and also normal hemoglobins A_2 and F (82,83). This is possible because there are enough structural differences between these Hbs and Hb A so that monospecific antibodies could be developed. However, the only difference between Hb A_o and Hb A_{Ic} is that in Hb A_{Ic} the β-chain NH_2 terminus has a hexose moiety attached to it. For this reason, it was not certain until 1978, when Javid et al. (84) demonstrated it, that a monospecific antibody could be prepared against Hb A_{Ic}. These investigators have produced antisera as follows: A cheviot sheep is injected biweekly with Hb A_{Ic} purified by Bio-Rex 70 chromatography. Each 5-ml injection contains 10 mg of Hb A_{Ic} in water and 2 ml of Freund's adjuvant. Each 5-ml injection is given at 25 intradermal sites. Following the eighth injection, 500 ml of blood are removed from the sheep on each nonimmunization week. The blood is left overnight at 4°C, and the serum is collected by centrifugation. The antiserum is repeatedly absorbed with agarose-linked Hb A_o to remove the cross-reacting antibodies, and the specificity of the residual antibodies for Hb A_{Ic} is monitored. Each antiserum is calibrated against the index antigen, namely, purified Hb A_{Ic} iodinated with ^{125}I by the chloramine-T method. A set of mixtures of purified Hb A_{Ic} and Hb A_o are used as the primary standards for the quantitative assay. For the assay, the reaction mixture, which contains 200 μl antiserum and 50 μl of hemoglobin (red cell hemolysate), is incubated at room temperature for 30 min. Index antigen is added to each reaction mixture and further incubated at room temperature for 30 min. The immune complex is precipitated with saturated ammonium sulfate, and the supernatant radioactivity is calculated from the counts in 1 ml and is expressed as the percent of total counts. Percentage blocking is defined as $(T-B)/(A-B) \times 100$ where T is the percent supernatant counts for test Hbs, A the antigen control, and B the antibody control. For assay purpose, a standard curve is constructed by plotting the percent blocking for each of the primary standards against its fractional content of Hb A_{Ic}. By reference to the standard curve, percent blocking values for the unknown is converted to percent Hb A_{Ic}.

Absorbing antiserum to Hb A_o-agarose improved the specificity of the antiserum to Hb A_{Ic}. However, this was achieved at the expense of considerable fall in antibody titer. Only about 10% of the initial titer was retained as specific anti-A_{Ic}. Hemoglobin A_o blocked the antiserum only minimally. Hemoglobin A_{Ia} and Hb A_{Ib} had 5 and 10% of the activity of Hb A_{Ic}, respectively, as judged by the quantities required for half-maximal blocking of the antiserum. In contrast, all fractions reacted equally well with the nonspecific anti-A. Glycosylated hemoglobins from other species also reacted with anti-A_{Ic} in a quantitatively similar manner as their human counterparts. Comparison of Hb A_{Ic} values by both the radioimmunoassay and the ion exchange method showed good correlation. The chief advantage of this method, apart from potential ease of application, rests in the ability of the method to measure Hb A_{Ic} in the presence of fetal hemoglobin. This method has not gained widespread recognition because a commercial assay is not yet available. Moreover, the relatively low titer for anti-A_{Ic} may be a reason for concern.

Another type of immunological procedure involves nephelometric quantitation of immune precipitants of Hb A_I and antibody (85). Rabbits are immunized with Hb A_{Ic}, and a nephelometer is used to quantitate Hb A_I. The antibody does not differentiate Hb A_I from Hb A_o. So, Hb A_I is first separated by column chromatography, and then the true level of Hb A_{Ic} in this fraction is determined nephelometrically after reaction with the antibody. The method correlates very well with the cation exchange short column chromatographic method.

VII. SPECTROPHOTOMETRIC METHOD

The spectrophotometric assay is based on the fact that organophosphorus compounds, such as 2,3-DPG and inositol hexaphosphate (phytic acid), bind to the N-terminal amino acids of the two β chains of hemoglobin A (86). This causes a conformational change of the hemoglobin molecule, a process that can be monitored spectrophotometrically. The spectrum of Hb A_{Ic} (Hb A_I, in general) will not change by organic phosphates because the N-terminus is already blocked. Thus, the change in absorbance induced by phytic acid is inversely proportional to the percentage of glycosylated hemoglobin.

For the spectrophotometric assay, a kit is available (Glycospec, Abbot Laboratories, North Chicago, Ill.) (86). An aliquot of each blood sample or standard is pipetted into sample cups. Ten microliters of each sample or Hb A_I standard are automatically dispensed with 500 μl of hemolyzing agent into the appropriate cuvette, and the difference in absorbance at 560 and 633 nm is recorded. Fifty microliters of phytic acid reagent are added into each cuvette, and the difference in abosrbance is again recorded. After correcting for total hemoglobin, the difference between the two readings is graphed against the percentage of Hb A_I in the standards. The percentage of Hb A_I in the blood samples may be obtained from the graph.

Both the spectrophotometric and ion exchange microcolumn methods had similar precision and reproducibility (86). However, the spectrophotometric method yielded consistently higher values than microcolumn methods; this is more evident in diabetics than in normals. The reason for this discrepancy has been postulated to be due to a competition between endogenous 2,3-DPG and phytic acids for the same binding sites in the hemoglobin molecule. In fact, exogenous 2,3-DPG causes a dose-related displacement of the standard curve. However, variations in the concentration of endogenous 2,3-DPG are not considered to influence significantly the Hb A_I values obtained with the spectrophotometric method. Even with whole blood levels of 1.6-2.8 mmol/liter of 2,3-DPG in diabetics, the difference in Hb A_I would only be about 0.5%. The Glycospec assay is sensitive to the anticoagulent used; heparin gives higher values than EDTA. Storage of blood samples at 22°C for a few days results in a sharp increase in Hb A_I with the Glycospec method. This is most likely due to denaturation of the hemoglobin, thus, affecting the phytic acid binding. The presence of Hb F, probably because of the inability of organic phosphates to bind to this hemoglobin, yields false increase in Hb A_I. Moreover, it is not known to what extent the labile Schiff base is measured by this approach. This spectrophotometric method appears to be less sensitive to small changes in temperature, pH, and ionic strength of the buffer, and the method can be automated for large-scale analysis.

VIII. COLORIMETRIC DETERMINATION—THIOBARBITURIC ACID (TBA) ASSAY

In 1976, Flückiger and Winterhalter (87) described an assay for glycosylated hemoglobin by estimating the hemoglobin-bound hexose. In this method, the hemoglobin-linked 2-ketoamine is converted to 5-hydroxymethylfurfural (5-HMF) (Fig. 4.29) by limited hydrolysis in a weak acid (oxalic acid). 5-Hydroxymethylfurfural forms a colored complex when reacted with thiobarbituric acid [(TBA), hence, TBA assay]. This complex absorbs between 400 and 480 nm, with a wavelength maximum of 443 nm. According to the original method employed by Flückiger and Winterhalter (87), 1 ml of 0.3 N oxalic acid is added

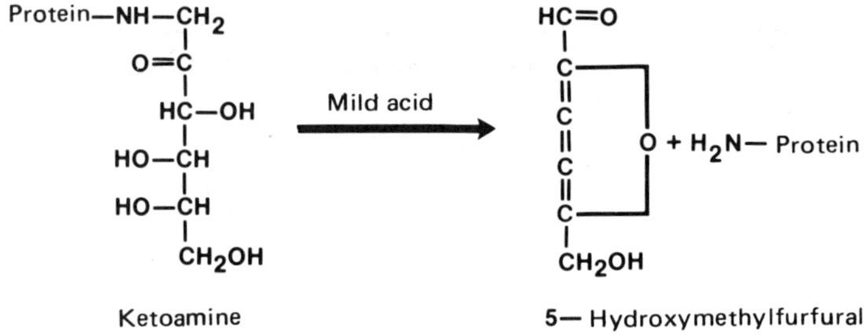

Figure 4.29 The conversion Hb (protein)-linked 2-ketohexose to 5-hydroxymethylfurfural (5-HMF) while heating with mild acid.

to 2 ml of hemolysate (10 g hemoglobin/dl), and the mixture is heated for 1 hr at 100°C. After cooling to room temperature, 1 ml of a trichloroacetic acid solution (40 g/dl) is added, the mixture is shaken, and then centrifuged for 10 min at 3000 rpm. Two milliliters of the supernatant are mixed with 0.5 ml of 0.05 M of TBA and incubated for 40 min at 40°C. Optical density is read at 443 nm. The percentages of Hb A_{Ic} in the samples are calculated based on the finding that 1% Hb A_{Ic} gives a TBA assay optical density reading of 0.029. This method, without much modifications, was applied for the quantitation of Hb A_{Ic}, and the correlation with the Hb A_{Ic} values obtained by the Bio-Rex 70 methods was generally poor (10). These data were obtained in a study of 48 patients with IDDM. From what is known now about the various sites of glycosylation, it is apparent that converting the TBA assay values to Hb A_{Ic} percentages may not be valid at all. Moreover, it seems that the amount of hemoglobin used for the assay is too large and the hydrolysis time is too short to achieve a complete release of the 5-HMF.

In a modified TBA assay, 1 ml of hemoglobin (150 μM in heme; 2.4 mg hemoglobin) is added to 0.5 ml of 1.0 N oxalic acid, and the mixture is heated at 100°C for 4 hr (7,88). The protein is then precipitated with 40% TCA and filtered through a 0.45 μ Millipore filter. One milliliter of the filtrate is mixed with the TBA reagent and incubated for 40 min at 40°C. The absorbances at 443 nm are used as such for quantitative evaluation of total glycohemoglobin. The results also may be expressed as A_{443} per milligram of hemoglobin. With this improvement, good correlation of the TBA assay values with Hb A_I values determined by a Bio-Rex 70 microcolumn method (Fig. 4.30) was observed with GHb values determined by affinity chromatography (Fig. 4.22) and with fluorometric glyco group analysis (see Fig. 4.30). Thus a reduction in the total hemoglobin used for the assay and an increase in the duration of the mold acid treatment have apparently increased the efficiency of the technique.

Subramanian et al. (89) modified the colorimetric assay by using globin preparations rather than hemoglobin. In this method, globin is made by adding 1 ml of hemolysate to 15 ml of cold acid-acetone. The optimum hydrolysis condition is 16 hr at 100°C in 10 mol/liter acetic acid. The formation and stability of the HMF-TBA color complex is maximal at 40°C and 50 min. Using the appropriate concentrations of 5-HMF standards, the results are expressed as HMF index, which is equal to micromoles of 5-HMF formed per gram of globin protein. The HMF index up to a value of 4.0 shows acceptable correlation with

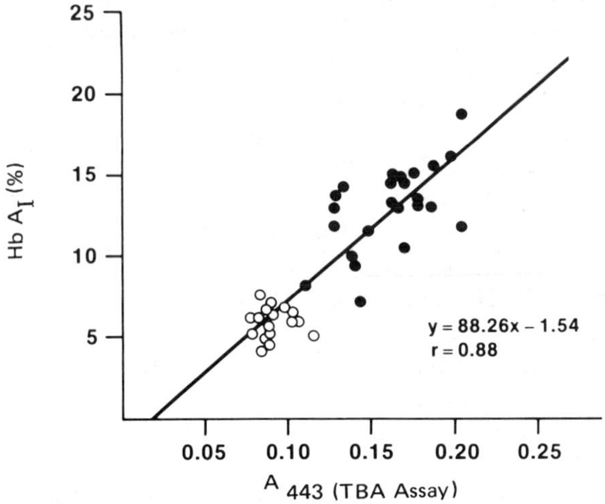

Figure 4.30 Correlation of TBA assay values (A_{443}) with percentage of Hb A_I in normals (○) and in diabetics (●).

Hb A_I values obtained by a commercial microcolumn assay. For higher index values, however, the correlation decreases. This is probably due to contribution from glycosylation of sites other than the β-chain NH_2 terminus. Improved correlation have been obtained with the levels of fasting blood sugar or mean fasting blood sugar (three or four measurements over the past 4 months) with 5-HMF index corrected for the mean hemoglobin concentration. This improved assay seems to be more sensitive than the procedure that uses oxalic acid for hydrolysis. The methodology, however, applied here appears to be more complicated and more time-consuming than the other conventional colorimetric methods and is somewhat less suitable for routine clinical laboratory work.

Parker et al. (90) modified the hydrolysis step by autoclaving with 0.5 M oxalic acid for 60 min at 124°C. This modification has considerably shortened the hydrolysis time and has enhanced the 5-HMF formation. The assay procedure adopted is as follows: Combine in screw-capped tubes (13 × 100 mm) with Teflon-lined caps, 1 ml of diluted hemoglobin (10 mg of hemoglobin) or fructose standard with 1 ml of oxalic acid reagent (0.5 mol/liter). Heat the tightly sealed tubes for 60 min in the autoclave at 124°C. After cooling to room temperature and mixing the contents by inversion, 1 ml of 40% trichloroacetic acid is added. The contents are again mixed and filtered through a 15 × 0.5 cm glass column with a glass wool plug in the bottom. To 1.5 ml of the filtrate, add 0.5 ml of 0.05 M thiobarbituric acid reagent. Incubate the tubes in a water bath at 40°C for 30 min, allow to cool to room temperature for 15 min, and measure the absorbance at 443 nm. In addition to the patients' samples (unknowns), each assay includes 40, 50, 60, 70, and 80 μmol/liter of fructose standards and control samples of normal hemolysate pool and diabetic hemolysate pool. For each hemolysate, an appropriate blank is prepared, merely omitting the final color development step with thiobarbituric acid. The absorbance at 443 nm of each blank is subtracted from that of the corresponding sample. For conversion of the measured absorbances for the hemolysates to nanomoles of 5-HMF, a relative absorptivity of 0.009 for the complex formed between 5-HMF and thiobarbituric acid is used. To convert absorbances to fructose equivalents, a fructose standard curve is used. Excellent within assay and between assay CVs have been reported for this modified TBA assay. Figure 4.31 gives a fructose standard curve, and Fig. 4.32 gives a 5-HMF standard curve obtained in our laboratory. Figure 4.33 gives the results of a study of normals and diabetic patients, where the results of the TBA, expressed as nanomoles of 5-HMF per 10 mg of Hb, are compared with Hb A_I values obtained by a microcolumn method.

Several variables, such as oxalic acid concentration, hydrolysis interval, 5-hydroxymethylfurfural destruction, extraneous glucose, and hemoglobin concentration, influence the extimation of glycosylated hemoglobin with this colorimetric method (7,89-92). Mild acid hydrolysis does not remove all of the hexose from its binding site. This may be especially true for Hb A_{Ia+b} and for those glycosylated hemoglobins formed by glycosylation at sites other than the β-chain amino terminus. However, stronger acid hydrolysis, to obtain more a complete release of the carbohydrate, increases the rate of 5-HMF destruction. Thus, the amount of 5-HMF assayed will reflect a smaller amount of sugar than actually is attached to the hemoglobins. Consequently, the measured 5-HMF will not be stoichiometrically related to glycosylated hemoglobin. However, such a relationship may not be essential to set up a reliable colorimetric assay if the assay conditions are well controlled and de-

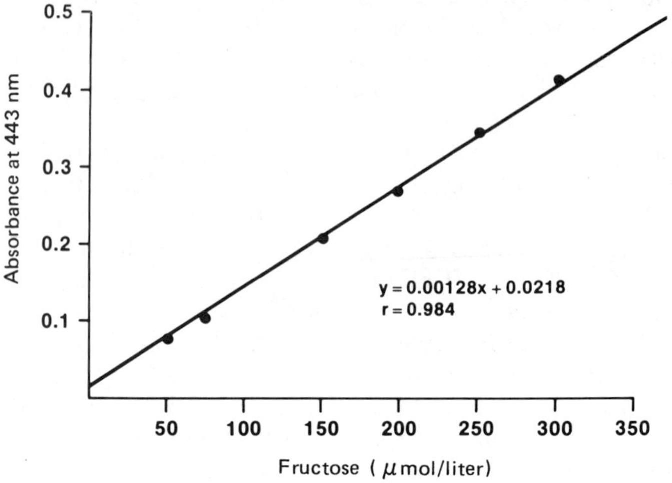

Figure 4.31 Fructose concentration dependence of the absorbance at 443 nm of the TBA-5-HMF complex.

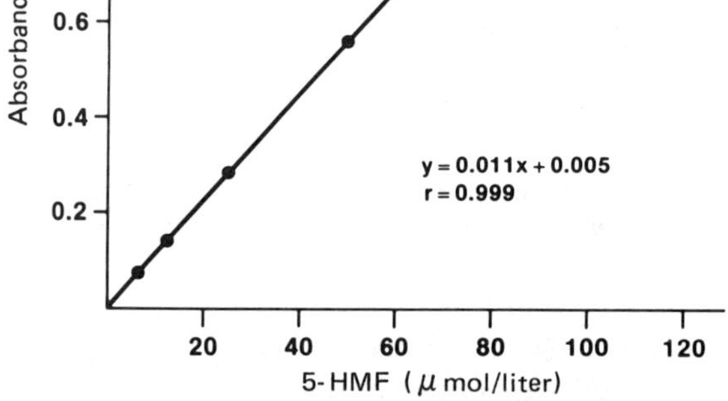

Figure 4.32 5-Hydroxymethylfurfural concentration dependence of the absorbance at 443 nm of the TBA-5-HMF complex.

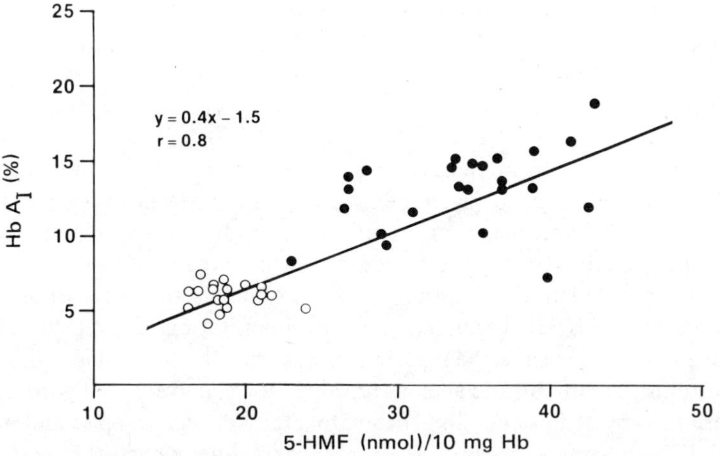

Figure 4.33 Correlation of the TBA assay values expressed as nanomoles of 5-HMF per 10 mg of Hb with the Hb A_I levels determined by a cation exchange microchromatographic method in normals (○) and in diabetics (●).

fined. Although the mechanism is not clear, abnormally high glucose soncentrations can influence the apparent 5-HMF levels. This interference by free glucose can vary from sample to sample, but can be eliminated by washing the red cells. Up to 30% of the 5-HMF may be destroyed during a 5-hr hydrolysis. This estimate, which is obtained by hydrolysis of added HMF in the presence of hemoglobin, may be too high because in the real assay conditions 5-HMF is only gradually produced during the entire hydrolysis period rather than being present as free 5-HMF even from the beginning. The rate of 5-HMF formation and destruction varies with the vigor of hydrolysis conditions, which must be adequately controlled with respect to temperature, acid concentration, and incubation time. Hemoglobin concentrations in blood samples also vary from sample to sample, thus requiring adjustment of the final hemoglobin concentration before hydrolysis or relying on a correction factor to compensate for deviations from the optimal protein concentrations. This step can be eliminated if the results are expressed as mole-percent. This is possible only because the rate of 5-HMF formation is not significantly influenced by the normal variations in hemoglobin concentration; no significant difference has been observed even at concentrations ranging from 15.5 to 31.0 g/dl. Nonspecific background color developing during the hydrolysis step is another possible interference in the colorimetric assay. Some laboratories have recommended using a blank for each sample. However, since this background is rather non-variable among specimens, including one sample in the assay and subtracting its absorbance value from the absorbance of each blood sample may be an easier approach.

Since it has undergone numerous improvements and extensive evaluations, the colorimetric assay for glycosylated hemoglobin has gained more acceptance and recognition as a reliable means of monitoring therapy in diabetic patients. The release of the hexose from glycosylated hemoglobin may not be complete, but with well-controlled assay conditions, it is reproducible and linear to high concentrations of glycosylated hemoglobin. The quantitation of glycosylated hemoglobins is possible even in the presence of abnormal hemoglobins and fetal hemoglobin. Thiobarbituric acid assay values correlate very well with GHb values determined by affinity column chromatography in such samples and in normal and diabetic samples as well. The presence of aldimine Schiff base should not interfere with this assay, since only the ketoamine can form 5-HMF, and thus only this form of the glycosylated hemoglobins is quantitated by this method. Extraordinary care in storage of the samples is not needed because formation of Hb A_{Id} due to in vitro aging should not affect the assay, except that storage conditions that denature hemoglobin should be avoided.

IX. FLUOROMETRIC DETERMINATION OF GLYCO GROUPS

Gallop et al. (93) have described a chemical method for determining protein glycosylation that is based on fluorometric determination of formaldehyde released by periodate oxidation of the carbohydrate moieties. Formaldehyde released upon periodate oxidation may derive either from the C-1 carbon of the 1-amino-1-deoxy-2-ketose or from the C-6 carbon of the 1-amino aldose. The resulting formaldehyde is quantitated as the fluorescent condensation product, 3,5-diacetyl-1,4-dihydrolutidine, formed with acetylacetone and ammonia (formaldehyde detection reagent) in the Hantzsch reaction. In this method, globin preparations rather than hemoglobin preparations are used. For preparation of globin, up to 1 ml of hemolysate is added dropwise to 10 ml of freshly prepared cold 1% tetrahydrofuran (THF) in 12 N hydrochloric acid. The precipitated globin is centrifuged and washed at least twice with cold THF. The THF is decanted, the protein is dissolved in 1 to 2 ml of water, and the optical density at 280 nm is recorded. The protein concentration is calculated based on the percent extinction coefficient $E_{1\%} = 8.5$. To 2-4 mg of protein in 700 μl of water are added 20 μl of 1 N HCl. Oxidation is started by the addition of 100 μl of 0.1 N $NaIO_4$ and is allowed to proceed at room temperature for 30 min. The samples are cooled on ice, and 300 μl of ice cold zinc sulfate and 100 μl of 1.4 N NaOH are added. This step will precipitate the excess periodate. The samples are then centrifuged, and the supernatant is collected. Following the addition of freshly prepared formaldehyde detection reagent (1 ml of 2 M ammonium acetate and 0.02 M of acetylacetone in water), the fluorescence is allowed to develop for 1 hr at 37°C. Fluorescence is measured by excitation at 410 nm and emission at 510 nm. Fructose standards (0-40 nmol) are simultaneously run with each assay. The number of nanomoles of fructose equivalents per milligram of globin is obtained from the standard curve and converted to glyco groups per αβ dimer using the formula: glyco groups/αβ dimer equals 0.032 × fructose equivalents (nmol) per mg globin, taking into consideration that the molecular weight of the αβ globin dimer is 32,000 and that one equivalent of formaldehyde is released from 1 mol of fructose and 1 equivalent of a ketoamine glyco group.

In order to quantitate hemoglobin glycosylation by periodate oxidation, it is necessary to remove all the periodate-sensitive formaldehyde-yielding compounds. This is achieved by preparing globin with acid THF, as hemin and acetone used in certain other procedures may interfere with the fluorometric assay. At acidic conditions (pH 3.0), periodate oxidation proceeds quickly and reaches completion in about 20 min. Although a final periodate concentration of 12.2 nM is used in the assay, it seems that concentrations between 1 to 30 mM can be used without affecting the release of formaldehyde. It is highly critical that the excess periodate is completely removed, otherwise this periodate could decrease the fluorescence yield. At low formaldehyde concentration, the condensation reaction with acetylacetone and ammonia is nearly quantitative in the pH range of 5.5-6.5. Formaldehyde release from the carbohydrate moieties increases linearly with protein concentration from 1 to 12 mg of globin, although analysis is usually done with 1 to 5 mg of globin. When a fructose standard curve is used, the slope of the standard curve is calculated from values up to 40 mmol of frustose because the fructose standard curve is nonlinear beyond this concentration.

The glyco group content of Hb A_{Ic} was shown to be 1.14 glyco groups per αβ dimer and of Hb A_o was 0.18. The value for Hb A_{Ic}, in which each β chain is N-terminally glycosylated, agrees well with the expected value. Acceptable correlations were obtained of the number of glyco groups with the levels of Hb A_I determined by cation exchange microcolumn chromatography (Fig. 4.34), GHb determined by affinity chromatography (Fig. 4.21), and ketoamine

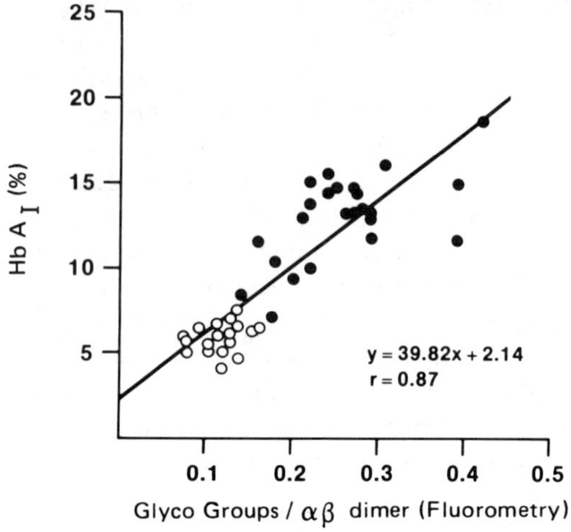

Figure 4.34 Correlation of the number of glyco groups determined fluorometrically with the Hb A_I levels in normals (○) and in diabetics (●).

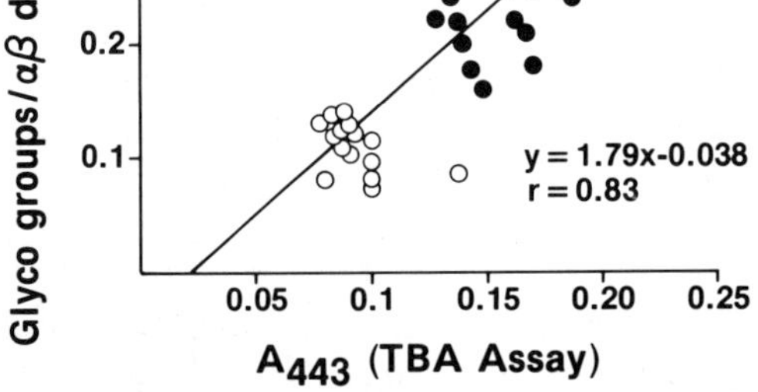

Figure 4.35 Correlation of the fluorometric assay for glyco groups with the colorimetric assay for ketoamine.

determined colorimetrically (Fig. 4.35). When hemolysate rich in Schiff base is analyzed by the fluorometric and ion exchange methods, increased number of glyco groups and increased Hb A_I values are observed, but no increases in GHb by the affinity method and HMF equivalents by the TBA assay. Thus, Schiff-base-linked glucose is measured by the fluorometric method. With the rapid automation, the fluorometric method may become practical for the routine analysis of clinical samples. Moreover, it is a rigorous method that precisely defines the total glyco group content of hemoglobin, rather than just the content of Hb A_I. The method may be adapted for the quantitation of nonenzymatic glycosylation of proteins that are otherwise enzymatically glycosylated or not. For estimation of nonenzymatic glycosylation in the presence of enzymatic glycosylation, prior reduction with $NaBH_4$ is essential. The difference in the amount of formaldehyde released from periodate oxidation of $NaBH_4$-reduced and unreduced proteins can measure the nonenzymatically produced ketoamine glyco groups (93).

X. COMMENTS

The preceding description of the various methods of quantitation of glycosylated hemoglobins provides the principles involved in each method in sufficient technical details and provides the limitations or advantages for routine clinical application. Macro- and microchromatographic methods utilizing the carboxylate resin Bio-Rex 70 or IRC-50 are still widely used for the separation and quantitation of glycosylated hemoglobin components A_{Ia+b} or A_{Ic} or the total Hb A_I. Provided that appropriate precautions are taken in controlling the chromatographic conditions, such as temperature and avoiding common interferences, such as Schiff-base aldimine, Hb F, and abnormal hemoglobins, ion exchange chromatography will continue to be a popular and reliable means of quantitating glycosylated hemoglobins. However, it should be pointed out that more recent studies involving affinity chromatographic and Bio-Rex 70 chromatographic separations of minor hemoglobins indicate that the true levels of Hb A_I may be overestimated by the ion exchange method. With affinity chromatography and chemical methods, an evaluation of the total glycosylated hemoglobin is possible. Moreover, the glycosylated hemoglobin levels determined by these methods are not influenced by those factors that influence glycosylated hemoglobin levels determined by ion exchange chromatography. It is not known whether determination of total glycosylated hemoglobin rather than Hb A_I or Hb A_{Ic} is of any special advantage in monitoring control of diabetes. The precision and reproducibility of the four

Table 4.11 Comparison of the Precision and Reproducibility of Glycosylated Hemoglobin Assay by Ion Exchange, Affinity, and Chemical Methods[a]

	Precision within run (CV)		Precision between run (CV)	
Methods of analysis	Normal sample (%)	Diabetic sample (%)	Normal sample (%)	Diabetic sample (%)
% Hb A_I (ion exchange)	0.5	0.8	1.8	2.2
% GHb (affinity)	1.5	1.0	5.3	3.8
A_{443} (TBA assay)	4.2	2.3	3.8	1.2
Glyco groups/$\alpha\beta$ dimer (fluorometry)	2.3	2.1	4.0	2.7

[a]Each sample was analyzed ten times within a run or ten times by separate runs.

Table 4.12 Comparison of the Mean, Standard Deviation, and Range of Glycosylated Hemoglobin Levels Determined by Ion Exchange, Affinity, and Chemical Methods in Normals and Diabetics

Method	Sample	Mean	Standard deviation	Range
Isolab Fast Hb Test System (% Hb A_I)	Normal	6.0	0.8	4.2-7.6
	Diabetic	13.0	2.6	9.4-18.9
Isolab Glyc-Affin System (% GHb)	Normal	6.3	0.6	5.0-7.4
	Diabetic	16.4	4.0	9.1-24.1
TBA assay (A_{443})	Normal	0.091	0.009	0.082-0.096
	Diabetic	0.160	0.025	0.127-0.204
Fluorometric procedure (Glyco groups/$\alpha\beta$ dimer)	Normal	0.117	0.023	0.076-0.136
	Diabetic	0.262	0.066	0.176-0.420

methods mentioned above are equally good (Table 4.11). The means, standard deviations, and ranges found in normals and in diabetics by analyzing each sample by the four different methods discussed here are given in Table 4.12. The data from all the four methods indicate a clear-cut separation of the diabetic patients from the normals. Agar gel electrophoresis and isoelectric focusing are attractive alternatives to ion exchange methods. Although both these methods are relatively more expensive and cumbersome, analysis of a large number of samples in batches should make them suited for routine use. The radioimmunoassay method is still not commercially available because of the difficulty in producing sufficient antiserum with relatively high titer. At present, affinity chromatography seems to be the simplest and the most reliable means of determining glycosylated hemoglobin. This method has wider application than most other methods.

LIST OF ABBREVIATIONS

CV	coefficient of variation
EDTA	ethylenediaminetetraacetic acid
HEPES	*N*-2-hydroxymethylpiperazine-*N*-2-ethanesulfonic acid
TEMED	*N,N,N′,N′*-tetramethylethylenediamine
THF	tetrahydrofuran
Tris	tris(hydroxymethyl)aminomethane
UV	ultraviolet

REFERENCES

1. D. W. Allan, W. A. Schroeder, and J. J. Balog, *J. Am. Chem. Soc., 80:* 1628 (1958).
2. E. C. Abraham, N. D. Cope, N. N. Braziel, and T. H. J. Huisman, *Biochim. Biophys. Acta, 577:* 159 (1979).
3. E. C. Abraham, M. Stallings, B. F. Cameron, and T. H. J. Huisman, *Biochim. Biophys. Acta, 625:* 109 (1980).
4. W. A. Schroeder and T. H. J. Huisman, *The Chromatography of Hemoglobin,* Marcel Dekker, New York (1980).
5. E. C. Abraham, M. Stallings, A. Abraham, and R. Clardy, *Biochim. Biophys. Acta, 744:* 335 (1983).
6. E. C. Abraham, B. F. Cameron, A. Abraham, and M. Stallings, *J. Lab. Clin. Med., 104:* 602 (1984).

7. M. J. McDonald, R. Shapiro, M. Bleichman, J. Soloway, and H. F. Bunn, *J. Biol. Chem., 253:* 2327 (1978).
8. E. C. Abraham, *Biochim. Biophys. Acta, 667:* 168 (1981).
9. L. A. Trivelli, H. M. Ranney, and H. T. Lai, *New Engl. J. Med., 284:* 353 (1971).
10. E. C. Abraham, T. A. Huff, N. D. Cope, J. B. Wilson, Jr., E. D. Bransome, Jr., and T. H. J. Huisman, *Diabetes, 27:* 931 (1978).
11. G. D. Efremov, T. H. J. Huisman, K. Bowman, R. N. Wrightstone, and W. A. Schroeder, *J. Lab. Clin. Med., 84:* 657 (1974).
12. P. A. M. Kynoch and H. Lehman, *Lancet,* July 2, p. 16 (1977).
13. M. B. Jones, R. D. Koler, and R. T. Jones, *Hemoglobin, 2:* 53 (1978).
14. R. E. Davis and D. J. Nicol, *Lancet, 2:* 350 (1978).
15. J. Chou, C. A. Robinson, Jr., and A. L. Siegel, *Clin. Chem., 24:* 1708 (1978).
16. F. Maquart, A. Randoux, J. P. Borel, J. P. Poynard, D. Malgrange, and M. Leutenegger, *Biomedicine, 29:* 208 (1978).
17. Y. Blouquit, C. Senan, and J. Rosa, *J. Chromat., 275:* 41 (1983).
18. W. Wajcman, B. Dastuge, and D. Labie, *Clin. Chim. Acta, 92:* 33 (1979).
19. M. A. Rosenthal, *Hemoglobin, 3:* 215 (1979).
20. M. Simon and J. Eissler, *Diabetes, 29:* 467 (1980).
21. L. A. Kaplan, D. Cline, P. Gartside, S. Burstein, M. Sperling, and E. A. Stein, *Clin. Chem., 28:* 13 (1982).
22. M. L. Delgado and I. E. Daza, *Clin. Chem., 27:* 358 (1981).
23. G. T. Hammons, K. Tunger, J. M. McDonald, and J. M. Ladenson, *Clin. Chem., 28:* 1775 (1982).
24. J. Jongeneel and M. Van Wissen, *Clin. Chem., 25:* 642 (1979).
25. D. Dix, P. Cohen, S. Kingsley, J. Senkbeil, K. Sexton, *Clin. Chem., 28:* 195 (1982).
26. E. C. Abraham, R. E. Perry, and M. Stallings, *J. Lab. Clin. Med., 102:* 187 (1983).
27. W. D. Hankins and L. A. Holladay, *Clin. Chim. Acta, 104:* 251 (1980).
28. P. A. Svendsen, J. S. Christiansen, A. R. Andersen, B. Welinder, and J. Nerup, *Lancet, 1:* 1142 (1979).
29. P. A. Svendsen, J. S. Christiansen, U. Svegaard, B. S. Welinder, and J. Nerup, *Diabetologia, 19:* 130 (1980).
30. H. B. Mortensen, *Sci. Tools, 27:* 21 (1980).
31. H. B. Mortensen, *J. Chromat., 182:* 325 (1980).
32. M. Stallings and E. C. Abraham, *Hemoglobin, 8:* 509 (1984).
33. P. Compagnucci, M. G. Cartechini, G. Bolli, P. DeFeo, F. Santeusanio, and P. Brunetti, *Diabetes, 30:* 607 (1981).
34. D. M. Nathan, E. S. Avezzano, and J. L. Palmer, *Diabetes, 30:* 700 (1981).
35. E. Bissé, W. Berger, and R. Flückiger, *Diabetes, 31:* 630 (1982).

36. M. H. Jonah, M. Trinh, and J. S. Kraus, *Clin. Chem., 28:* 1250 (1982).
37. J. S. Kraus and M. H. Jonah, *Clin. Chem., 28:* 1395 (1982).
38. M. H. Jonah, J. S. Kraus, and P. G. Mohorn, *Clin. Chem., 29:* 1444 (1983).
39. J. S. Kraus, M. H. Jonah, S. C. Yau, and M. Trinh, *Clin. Chem., 29:* 713 (1983).
40. H. Aleyassine, *Clin. Chem., 25:* 1484 (1979).
41. R. E. Bernstein, *Clin. Chem., 26:* 174 (1980).
42. T. Kruiswijk, D. P. Diaz, and H. C. Holtkamp, *Clin. Chem., 27:* 642 (1981).
43. I. M. Klotz and J. W. O. Tam, *Proc. Natl. Acad. Sci., USA, 70:* 1313 (1973).
44. K. R. Bridges, G. J. Schmidt, M. Jensen, A. Cerami, and H. F. Bunn, *J. Clin. Invest., 56:* 201 (1975).
45. D. M. Nathan, T. B. Francis, and J. L. Palmer, *Clin. Chem., 29:* 466 (1983).
46. A. F. Caspari and K. Miedema, *Lancet, 2:* 758 (1977).
47. G. Schernthauer, K. H. Stummvoll, and M. D. Muller, *Lancet, 1:* 774 (1979).
48. E. T. Sawadu, Jr. and A. Virji, *Dialysis Transplant, 9:* 360 (1980).
49. M. J. deBoer, K. Miedema, and A. F. Caspari, *Diabetologia, 18:* 437 (1980).
50. K. G. Stanton, R. Davis, and J. Richmond, *Lancet, 1:* 100 (1978).
51. R. Flückiger, W. Harmon, M. Werner, S. Loo, and K. H. Gabbay, *New Engl. J. Med., 304:* 823 (1981).
52. V. J. Stevens, W. J. Fantl, C. B. Newman, R. V. Sims, A. Cerami, and C. M. Petersen, *J. Clin. Invest., 76:* 361 (1981).
53. K. K. Tsuboi, D. J. Thompson, E. M. Rush, and H. C. Schwartz, *Hemoglobin, 5:* 241 (1981).
54. E. C. Abraham, M. Stallings, A. Abraham, and G. J. Garbutt, *Biochim. Biophys. Acta, 705:* 76 (1982).
55. T. H. J. Huisman, J. B. Henson, and J. B. Wilson, *J. Lab. Clin. Med., 102:* 163 (1983).
56. D. Dix, P. Cohen, S. Kingsley, M. J. Lea, J. Senkbeil, and K. Sexton, *Clin. Chem., 25:* 494 (1979).
57. A. M. Dozy and T. H. J. Huisman, *J. Chromatogr., 40:* 62 (1969).
58. C. A. Gruber and M. D. Koetz, *Clin. Chem., 25:* 1970 (1979).
59. R. S. Schifreen, J. M. Hickinbotham, and G. N. Bowers, Jr., *Clin. Chem., 26:* 406 (1980).
60. J. E. Davis, J. M. McDonald, and L. Jarett, *Diabetes, 27:* 102 (1978).
61. R. A. Cole, J. S. Soeldner, P. J. Dunn, and H. F. Bunn, *Metabolism, 27:* 289 (1978).
62. P. J. Dunn, R. A. Cole, and J. S. Soeldner, *Metabolism, 28:* 777 (1979).

63. E. C. Abraham, A. Abraham, and M. Stallings, *J. Lab. Clin. Med.* (in press).
64. W. H. Weibers and P. Gilham, *Biochemistry, 9:* 4396 (1970).
65. A. K. Mallia, G. T. Hermanson, R. I. Krohn, E. K. Fujimoto, and P. K. Smith, *Anal. Lett., 14:* 649 (1981).
66. P. D. G. Dean, *Diabetologia, 21:* 579 (1981).
67. V. Bouriotis, J. Stott, and A. Galloway, *Diabetologia, 21:* 579 (1981).
68. D. C. Klenk, G. T. Hermanson, R. I. Krohn, E. K. Fugimoto, A. K. Mallia, P. K. Smith, J. D. England, M. W. Hsiao, R. R. Little, and D. E. Goldstein, *Clin. Chem.*, 2088 (1982).
69. E. C. Abraham, M. Stallings, A. Abraham, and M. M. Elseweidy, *Hemoglobin, 7:* 449 (1983).
70. M. M. Elseweidy and E. C. Abraham, *Am. J. Hemat., 16:* 375 (1984).
71. R. C. Allen, M. Stastny, D. Hallett, and M. A. Simmons, in *Electrophoresis,* (B. J. Radola, ed.), pp. 663, deGruyter, New York, (1980).
72. L. Menard, M. E. Dempsey, L. A. Blankstein, H. Alleyassine, M. Wacks, and J. S. Soeldner, *Clin. Chem., 26:* 1598 (1980).
73. H. Aleyassine, R. J. Gardiner, L. A. Blankstein, and M. E. Dempsye, *Clin. Chem., 27:* 472 (1981).
74. H. Svensson, *Arch. Biochem. Biophys., 132* (suppl. 1): 132 (1962).
75. J. W. Drysdale, P. Righetti, and H. F. Bunn, *Biochim. Biophys. Acta, 229:* 42 (1971).
76. P. Basset, Y. Beuzard, M. C. Garel, and J. Rosa, *Blood, 51:* 971 (1978).
77. K. M. Spicer, R. C. Allen, and M. G. Buse, *Diabetes, 27:* 384 (1978).
78. L. Beccaria, C. Giuseppe, E. Gianazza, B. Luppis, and P. G. Righetti, *Am. J. Hemat., 4:* 376 (1978).
79. H. B. Mortensen, *Sci. Tools, 27:* 21 (1980).
80. H. B. Mortensen, *J. Chromat., 182:* 325 (1980).
81. B. S. Welinder and P. A. Svendsen, *Diabetologia, 19:* 465 (1980).
82. F. A. Garver, M. B. Baker, C. S. Jones, M. Gravely, G. Altay, and T. H. J. Huisman, *Science, 196:* 1334 (1977).
83. F. A. Garver, M. B. Baker, and H. E. Grenett, *Biochim. Biophys. Acta, 624:* 28 (1980).
84. J. Javid, P. K. Pettis, R. J. Koenig, and A. Cerami, *Br. J. Haemat., 38:* 329 (1978).
85. P. P. Chou, J. Kerkay, and M. K. Gupta, *Anal. Lett., 14:* 1071 (1981).
86. O. Walinder, G. Rouquist, and P. Fager, *Clin. Chem., 28:* 96 (1982).
87. R. Flückiger and K. H. Winterhalter, *FEBS Lett., 71:* 356 (1976).
88. J. Solway, M. McDonald, H. F. Bunn, F. Aun, R. Cole, and J. S. Soeldner, *J. Lab. Clin. Med., 93:* 962 (1979).
89. C. V. Subramanian, B. Radhakrishnamurthy, and G. S. Berenson, *Clin. Chem., 20:* 1083 (1980).

90. K. M. Parker, J. D. England, J. D. Costa, R. L. Hess, and D. E. Goldstein, *Clin. Chem., 27:* 669 (1981).
91. R. E. Pecoraro, R. J. Grag, J. B. Halter, H. Beiter, and D. Porte, Jr., *Diabetes, 27:* 1120 (1979).
92. K. H. Gabbay, J. M. Sosenko, G. A. Banuchi, M. J. Minisohn, and R. Flückiger, *Diabetes, 28:* 337 (1979).
93. P. M. Gallop, R. Flückiger, A. Hanneken, M. M. Mininsohn, and K. H. Gabbay, *Anal. Biochem., 117:* 427 (1981).

5

Clinical Relevance of Glycosylated Hemoglobins

I. GLYCOSYLATED HEMOGLOBINS IN DIABETES

A. Glycosylated Hemoglobin for Monitoring Glucose Control and Assessing Clinical Management of Diabetes

For almost 50 years, since insulin therapy was initiated, proponents of rigid or chemical control of hyperglycemia have quoted retrospective evidence of decreased or delayed complications as glucose levels are brought toward the normal range (1). Experimental evidence and recent studies employing insulin infusion pumps and home blood glucose monitoring have reported improvements in the parameters associated with microvascular complications (1-5). Proof that near-euglycemia prevents the development of microvascular complication awaits further study. However, in a small study of randomly assigned patients reported from Paris (6), patients with well-controlled diabetes showed less retinopathy. Thus, it is strongly believed that "good" or "better" control, when achievable, is beneficial. A major problem of previous studies has been the lack of an acceptable definition of "good" control." Previous criteria for assessing glycemic control have primarily relied upon spot urine testing for glucose, 24-hr measurements of

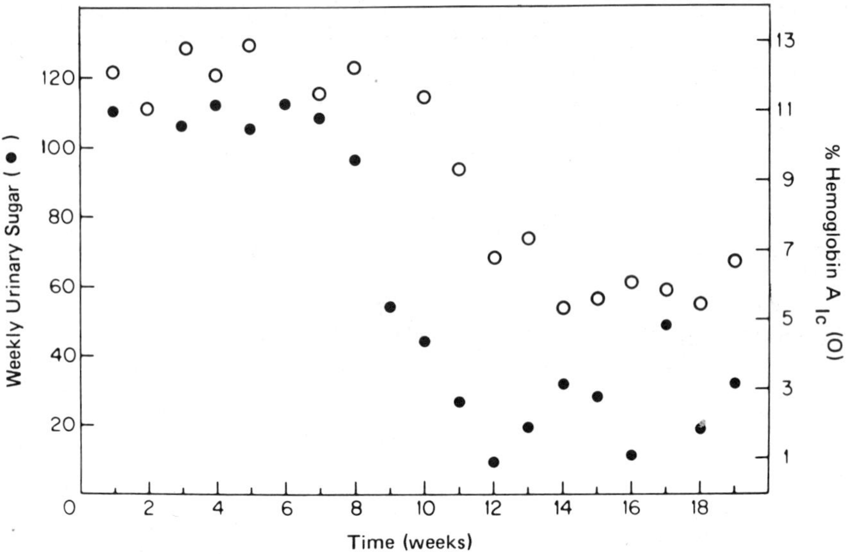

Figure 5.1 Temporal relation between weekly urinary sugar (●) and hemoglobin A_{Ic} (○) in a patient with type I diabetes. From Koenig et al. (7) by permission of the *New England Journal of Medicine.*

urine glucose, and sporadic blood sugar determinations. Urine glucose assessment has been the main tool in the day-to-day assessment of glycemic control. Urine glucose measurements, however, are at best qualitative and may not correlate well with simultaneous blood slucose analysis. A new approach, namely, glycosylated hemoglobin assay, is considered to be a better tool to assess blood glucose control.

A series of studies done during the latter part of the 1970s and some done more recently have confirmed the utility of Hb A_{Ic}, Hb A_I, or GHb measurement as a monitor of glucose control in patients with IDDM (type I diabetes) and non-insulin-dependent diabetes mellitus (NIDDM) or type II diabetes. It was demonstrated in 1976 by Koenig et al. (7) that when patients with type I diabetes were brought under control in the hospital, it took 8 to 12 weeks for their glycosylated hemoglobin levels to return to normal (Figs. 5.1 and 5.2). Thus, the concept that single Hb A_{Ic} determination reflects the time-averaged serum glucose concentration for the preceding 8 to 12 weeks was established. The temporal relation between the decrease in Hb A_{Ic} con-

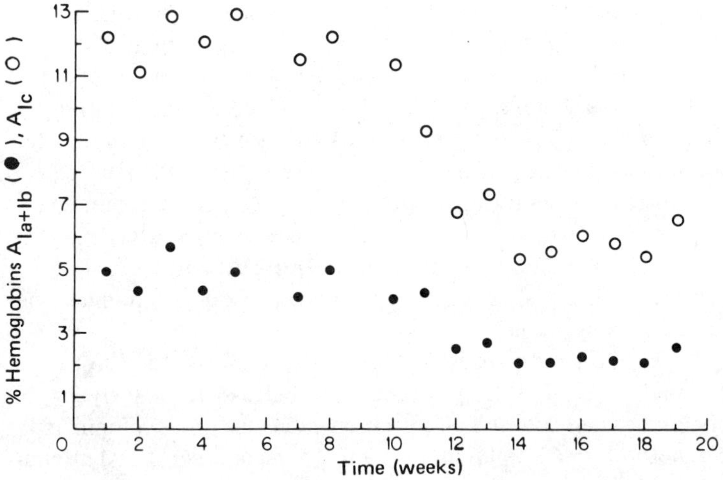

Figure 5.2 Temporal relation between the levels of hemoglobins A_{Ia+b} (●) and A_{Ic} (○) in a diabetic patient. From Koenig et al. (7) by permission of the *New England Journal of Medicine.*

centration and improved carbohydrate metabolism was clear-cut as judged by weekly summation of semiquantitative urinary sugar determination (Fig. 5.1). The decrease in urinary sugar preceded the change in Hb A_{Ic} concentration by approximately 3-4 weeks. The change in the concentration of Hb A_{Ia+b}, although smaller in absolute amount, occurred at the same time as the decrease in Hb A_{Ic} levels (Fig. 5.2). Hemoglobin A_{Ic} levels correlated not only with the steady state but also with the transient states during the process of improving serum glucose values. This has been established by the observation that both glycosuria and six serial serum glucose determinations made throughout the day around mealtimes have correlated with Hb A_{Ic} concentrations. Similar results have been reported in an outpatient setting in which glucose normalization process may take longer (8). Hemoglobin A_{Ic} was measured at the start of an insulin therapy program aided by home glucose monitoring. The mean Hb A_{Ic} concentration was 10.3% at the beginning of the program, and it decreased to a plateau 6 weeks into the program, thus reflecting the time course necessary to normalize serum glucose concentration.

Gonen et al. (9) found close correlation of the physicians' ratings of the degree of control and fasting plasma glucose levels with Hb A_I levels in ambulatory diabetic patients. The degree of control of 72 diabetic patients was rated by their clinic physicians on a scale of 1 to 5, 1 being defined as extremely poor, 2 as moderately poor, 3 as fair, 4 as good, and 5 as excellent. In this study, the various expressions of the plasma glucose concentration, namely, fasting plasma glucose (single measurement or mean of several daily values), mean of daily plasma glucose levels, and the highest daily glucose concentration, correlated significantly with Hb A_I levels. These results suggest that Hb A_I level is a useful indicator of the degree of hyperglycemia that exists over long periods. Good correlation between Hb A_I and the fasting glucose concentration is not always found in a diabetic population unless the diabetic state is relatively stable.

In 1977, we conducted a study to assess the suitability of Hb A_I or Hb A_{Ic} determination in monitoring control of diabetes (10). The glycosylated hemoglobins were determined by cation exchange microcolumn and macrocolumn methods in 61 children, ages 9 to 15 years, with IDDM attending a 2-week-long diabetic camp. Each child brought to the camp a dossier describing his own physician's evaluation of the control of his diabetes for the previous 3-6 weeks. Criteria of the management of diabetes were applied without prior knowledge of the glycosylated hemoglobin values. A score of 1 to 5 was assigned to each person, a score of 1 indicating poor management of control, and a score of 5 indicating good management. The data used were blood and urinary glucose records from the 3 months preceding the camp and during the camp, when available; records from the prior year; an evaluation by the patient's family physician of exceptionally good or poor control; and observations of the acceptance of diabetes management techniques by the patient and family as noted by the family physician and his associates and by the teaching nurses and staff physicians at the diabetic camp. Rather significant information was obtained when the Hb A_I values obtained by micro- and macrocolumn methods and Hb A_{Ic} levels determined by macrochromatography in the diabetic children were divided among the five management groups (Figs. 5.3 and 5.4). It is noteworthy that the concentrations of the glycosylated hemoglobins are decreased in patient groups showing the better management ratings. There is considerable overlap in the Hb A_I or the Hb A_{Ic} values between the different groups, except for the values of group 1 (poor control) and those of the normal controls (group 6). The correlation of Hb A_I levels with the different management groups was similar to that of Hb A_{Ic} levels, indicating that assay for total Hb A_I rather than Hb A_{Ic} may be just enough for monitoring diabetic patients. The correlation between patient management groups and Hb A_I concentrations determined by the colorimetric pro-

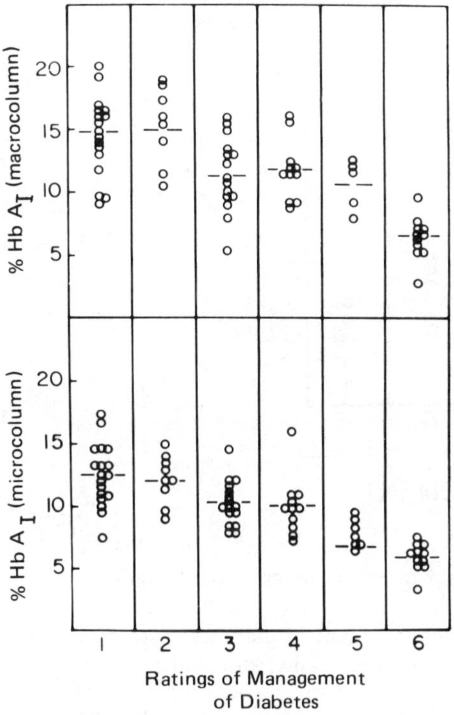

Figure 5.3 The levels of Hb A_I determined by both cation exchange microchromatography (the Isolab Fast Hemoglobin Test System) and macrochromatography (the Trivelli method) in 61 children with insulin-dependent diabetes mellitus, who had varying degrees of management of their diabetes. A score of 1 to 5 was assigned to each person, a score of 1 indicating poor management of control and a score of 5 indicating good management of control. Group 6 were normal controls. From Abraham et al. (10) by permission of the American Diabetes Association.

cedure of Flückiger and Winterhalter was decidedly poor. However, there is no reason to believe that with the application of improved colorimetric methods better correlation will not be observed. Since 1977, the commercially available microcolumns have undergone careful scrutiny, and several changes in the techniques have been introduced to assure improved reproducibility and precision. Moreover, in the meanwhile an affinity chromato-

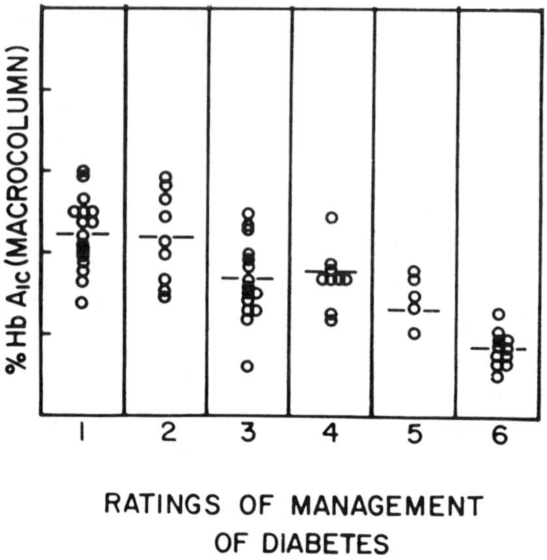

Figure 5.4 The levels of Hb A_{Ic} determined by macrochromatography (the Trivelli method) in 61 children with insulin-dependent diabetes mellitus arranged according to the ratings of management of diabetes; also see Fig. 5.3. From Abraham et al. (10) by permission of the American Diabetes Association.

graphic method has been developed to quantitate total glycosylated hemoglobin (GHb). In a more recent study conducted by us of another 43 children where the patient groups were arranged according to control ratings, both the Hb A_I and the GHb levels showed reduction that corresponded to successive improvements in control (Fig. 5.5 and Table 5.1). The GHb values seem to provide the best inverse relationship to the ratings of management of diabetes. In another study (11), control of diabetes was assessed during an 8-week camp program in 18 insulin-dependent patients with a mean age of about 19 years and a mean duration of diabetes of 11.4 years. A composite score was obtained from each subject on the basis of percent sugar-free urine tests, 24-hr glucose excretion as percent of carbohydrate uptake, and mean preprandial blood glucose. Scores ranging from 24 (fair control) to 45 (excellent control) showed a significant inverse correlation with Hb A_{Ic} and mean preprandial blood glucose. The Hb A_{Ic} was better predicted by percent sugar-free urine tests than by the 24-hr glucose excretion.

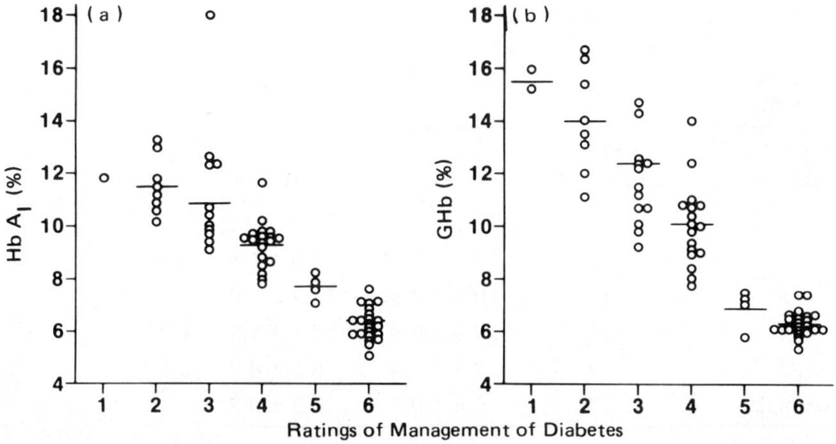

Figure 5.5 The levels of Hb A_I and GHb (determined by affinity chromatography) in 43 children with insulin-dependent diabetic children, the data being arranged according to the ratings of management of diabetes.

Davis et al. (12) showed that the mean Hb A_I levels measured in 186 diabetic patients and 108 nondiabetic controls were 7.45 ± 0.73% in the controls, 10.7 ± 0.2% in well-controlled diabetics, and 15.0 ± 2.5% in poorly controlled diabetics. Moreover, in patients with the onset of diabetes after the age of 40 years, there was a significant difference between the Hb A_I levels in those with diabetic retinopathy and in those without any such complications. There was significant association between Hb A_I levels and the duration of the disease in diabetes controlled with insulin. Ditzel and Kjaergaard (13) determined glycosylated hemoglobin components A_{Ia+b} and A_{Ic} serially in ten consecutive cases of newly discovered nonacidotic diabetic patients before and after diet and insulin treatment. The average concentration of Hb A_{Ic} was 11.4% in untreated diabetics, and, with prolonged optimal regulation of blood glucose Hb A_{Ic}, the average slowly decreased to a mean concentration of 5.5%. The return to normal values took from 25 to 80 days, and the rate of this return was dependent on the initial Hb A_{Ic} concentration and the degree of plasma glucose control. Jackson and co-workers (14) also noted a rapid decrease in Hb A_{Ic} levels to near normal values after type I diabetic patients were maintained euglycemic for 60 days. Gabbay et al. (15) found good correlation with glucose control as evaluated by urinary glucose assay performed 6 weeks prior to Hb A_{Ic} assay.

Table 5.1 Levels of Hb A_I and Total Glycosylated Hemoglobin (GHb) in Diabetic Patients Who Had Varying Degrees of Management and Control of Diabetes

Physicians'[a] ratings	Number of patients	Hb A_I (%)	GHb (%)
1	2	11.7	15.6
2	8	11.5 ± 1.0[b]	14.0 ± 1.8
3	12	10.9 ± 2.3	12.4 ± 3.4
4	17	9.3 ± 0.9	10.1 ± 1.5
5	4	7.7 ± 0.4	6.9 ± 0.7
Normals	25	6.4 ± 0.7	6.3 ± 0.5

[a]Rating 1 indicates poor and 5 indicates good management and control of diabetes.
[b]Mean ± S.D.

Dunn and co-workers (16) also found that in type I diabetics Hb A_I concentration was representative of the average degree of glycemia present during the 4-8 weeks prior to obtaining the sample. The same group also provided the first evidence that a single Hb A_{Ic} determination in a 3-month period is adequate for measure of diabetic control when the subjects are on a stable therapeutic regimen (17).

Although glycosylated hemoglobin accurately reflects the mean plasma glucose during the preceding weeks to months, a relationship between glycosylated hemoglobin levels and fasting plasma glucose concentration is not always seen (10). It may depend on the technique used for glycosylated hemoglobin assay and whether the parients are stable or unstable diabetics. Goldstein and co-workers (18) analyzed nearly 1200 paired Hb A_{Ic} and plasma glucose values (both fasting and 2-hr postprandial) in 187 youths (type I diabetic). The results indicated highly significant relationship between Hb A_{Ic} and both the fasting and 2-hr postprandial plasma glucose levels (Fig. 5.6). Similar data were also obtained by comparing Hb A_{Ic} levels to mean blood glucose levels resulted from home glucose monitoring. These authors also reported a statistically significant relationship between glycosylated hemoglobin levels and both duration of diabetes and insulin dose per kilogram body weight. In the patients they studied, insulin requirements rose gradually with the duration of diabetes and reached a

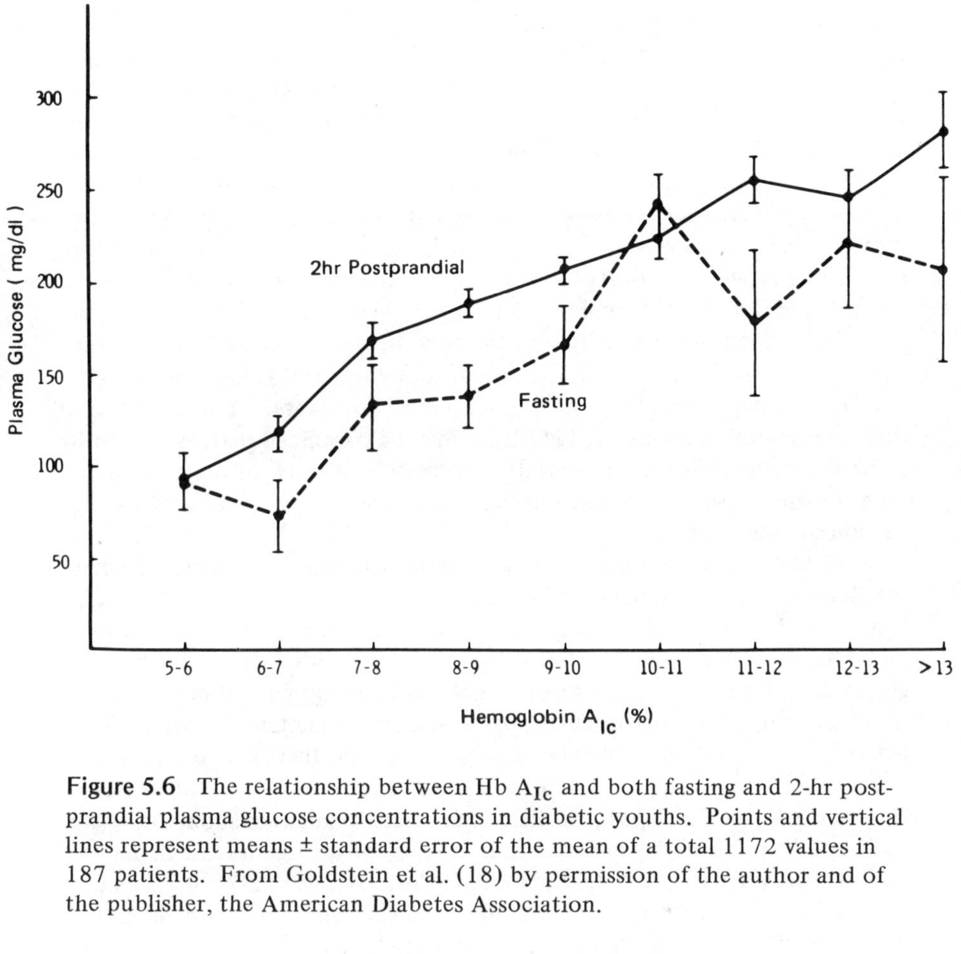

Figure 5.6 The relationship between Hb A_{Ic} and both fasting and 2-hr postprandial plasma glucose concentrations in diabetic youths. Points and vertical lines represent means ± standard error of the mean of a total 1172 values in 187 patients. From Goldstein et al. (18) by permission of the author and of the publisher, the American Diabetes Association.

plateau by 2-3 years duration. Interestingly, this increase paralleled the increase in glycosylated hemoglobin and the loss of endogenous insulin secretion.

The usefulness of glycosylated hemoglobin determinations to assess control of type II diabetic patients was evaluated by various investigators. Clarke (19) studied patients maintained on sulfonylurea compounds. The correlation between Hb A_I levels and fasting serum glucose was excellent in both mild and severe type II diabetics. This is in striking contrast with the generally observed relatively poor correlation between these two parameters in type I diabetic subjects. These differences may be explained by the relatively stable nature of glycemia in subjects with type II diabetics and the labile nature in type I diabetics. Boden et al. (20) investigated 15 type II diabetic patients receiving chlorpropamide therapy. The Hb A_{Ic} concentrations showed little fluctuation and accurately reflected the degree of control. Interestingly, when the therapy was withdrawn, the fasting serum glucose concentration increased, followed by an increase in Hb A_I within 1 week. Hemoglobin A_I levels continued to increase until a stable plateau was reached in about 3 weeks. After the oral hypoglycemic agent has been reinstituted, the fasting serum glucose concentration decreased from 180 to 140 mg/dl within the first week. Hemoglobin A_{Ic}, on the other hand, decreased gradually over the next 4-6 weeks. Thus, it is apparent that even in this in vivo setting, the rate of formation or the "on" rate for glycosylation is more rapid than the degradation or "off" rate. Thus, as a result of these and several other studies (21,22), it may be concluded that, as in type I diabetic patients, Hb A_{Ic} concentration accurately reflects glucose control in type II diabetic patients as well and that it is a useful clinical tool with which to monitor glucose control.

Goldstein and his associates made a serious attempt to understand what the glycosylated hemoglobin level means to a physician, and how he can realistically use this to treat diabetic patients (18). The conclusions made by this group have resulted from their long-time experience with glycosylated hemoglobin assay for monitoring control of diabetes in a large patient population. Ideally, an important diabetes care goal would be to maintain glycosylated hemoglobin levels in the nondiabetic range. However, there are doubts concerning whether such a goal is indeed realistic. Relative frequency distribution of Hb A_{Ic} and 2-hr postprandial plasma glucose values in about 200 diabetic youths participating in a longitudinal study of vascular disease in diabetes are provided in Fig. 5.7. The mean Hb A_{Ic} level was $9.37 \pm 0.2\%$ and 82% of values were less than 11%. Only four of the patients, however, had Hb A_{Ic} levels within the normal range. The results suggest that normalization of glycosylated hemoglobin levels may not be a realistic care goal in diabetic patients treated with conventional therapies. Even using the newer treatment approaches, such as subcutaneous insulin infusion pumps, normalization of the glycosylated hemoglobin is infrequently achieved, although the mean level is slightly lower than in patients treated with conventional insulin therapy. Therefore, a realistic and reasonable goal for blood glucose control would be to lower the expectations and set Hb A_{Ic} level at a slightly higher than normal level, say 9%. This corresponds to a Hb A_{Ia+b} level of about 10%. This is a justifiable approach because only a few patients could achieve and maintain

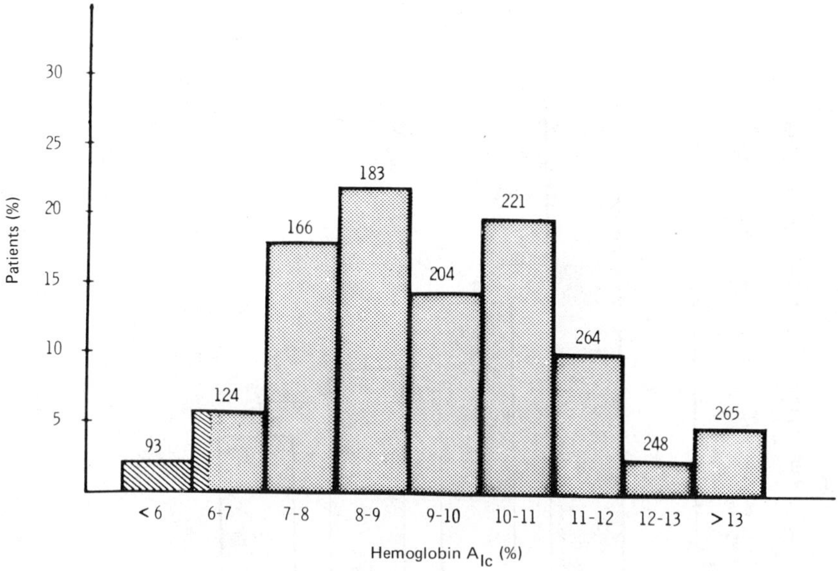

Figure 5.7 Frequency distribution of Hb A_{Ic} values in 187 patients with insulin-dependent diabetes mellitus. Numbers over vertical bars show the mean 2-hr postprandial plasma glucose concentrations in mg/dl for each of the Hb A_{Ic} categories. From Goldstein et al. (18) by permission of the author and of the American Diabetes Association.

Hb A_{Ic} levels in the nondiabetic range. In fact, patients with normal or nearly normal levels of glycosylated hemoglobin are at a much more increased risk of experiencing serious symptomatic hypoglycemia than those with moderately high levels of glycosylated hemoglobin (Fig. 5.8). For these reasons, more modest goals that are more easily achievable were adopted by the authors. Glycosylated hemoglobin may be successfully used as an educational and diabetic care reinforcement tool. In this program, patients and their families are instructed in the advantages and disadvantages of the methods that are available to assess blood glucose control. Glycosylated hemoglobins are presented to the health professionals and the patients as an index of blood glucose control over an extended period of time. The measurement of glycosylated hemoglobins, however, does not replace home urine and blood glucose monitoring, which provide important information for day-to-day care decision. At each clinic

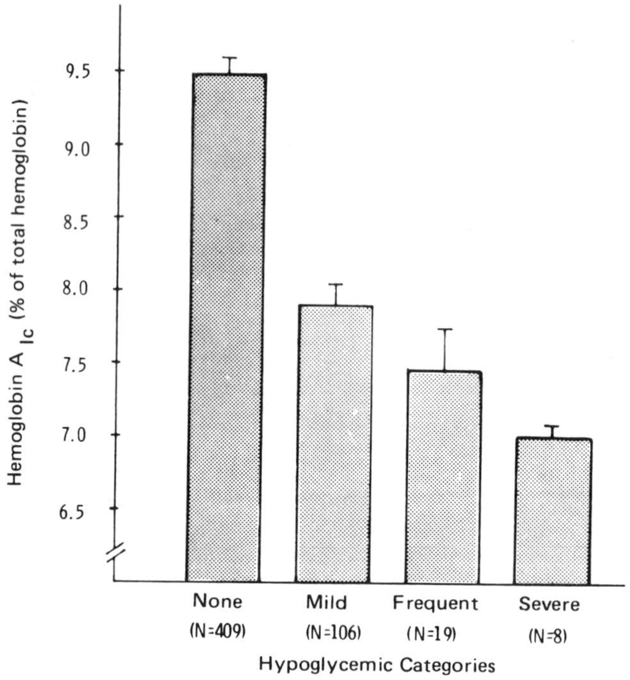

Figure 5.8 The relationship between Hb A_{Ic} and symptomatic hypoglycemia. Vertical bars and lines represent mean ± standard error of mean of a total of 542 values in 147 diabetic patients. At each clinic visit, patients were separated into one of four hypoglycemic categories based on the medical history since the preceding visit: no hypoglycemic reactions (none); mild to occasional reactions (mild); mild to frequent reactions (frequent); or severe reactions (severe). From Goldstein et al. (18) by permission of the author and of the American Diabetes Association.

visit, patients receive letters that include a report of their Hb A_{Ic} analysis and a brief note discussing the test results. The results of Hb A_{Ic} tests are displayed as a hemoglobin A_{Ic} "meter" to give the patient and family a better appreciation of what the test results mean. To increase patient interest in the use of glycosylated hemoglobin to monitor glucose control, when the patient complies with the treatment regimen as evidenced by an acceptable level of Hb A_{Ic}, 9% or under, he is invited to join a "club," i.e., the "Under Nine Club." However, it must be emphasized that it is an arbitrary decision to set a Hb A_{Ic} goal of 9%, and it cannot be universally applied; each diabetes care program must develop its own set of goals based on its specific treatment approach and the characteristics of the patient population.

The actual variability of glycosylated hemoglobin levels with brief periods of poor control have been questioned. The problem could be simply due to the presence of aldimine Schiff base, which in most instances is responsible for the fluctuations in Hb A_I or Hb A_{Ic}. However, employing an aldimine elimination step or choosing an appropriate method that quantitates only the ketoamine are the necessary steps for improving clinical correlation of glycosylation assay. Although glycosylated hemoglobin determinations are useful in assessing average glycemic control, individual monitoring of daily blood glucose is required for the daily management of diabetic patients.

B. Glycosylated Hemoglobin: A Genetic Marker or an Index of Metabolic Control

Soon after the discovery of Hb A_{Ic} and its elevation in patients with diabetes mellitus, two possibilities were brought up to explain this. It might represent a distorted carbohydrate metabolism or be an inherited component of the diabetic syndrome. To find out whether an increase in Hb A_{Ic} is due to an acquired or genetic abnormality, a study of identical twins concordant and discordant for diabetes was initiated by Tattersal et al. (23). The mean values for the proportion of Hb A_I in discordant twins differed markedly in two members of the pair. In concordant twins with type I diabetes, no marked differences in Hb A_I were observed between members of twin pairs. Four pairs of identical twins concordant for type II diabetes showed lower mean values for Hb A_I, but did not show marked intrapair differences. Thus, it appeared that the elevated level of glycosylated hemoglobin has no direct genetic basis but is a manifestation of metabolic abnormality of diabetes. Similar conclusions could be made based on the studies conducted on genetically induced diabetic mice, nondiabetic mice, and chemically induced diabetic mice (23). Genetically induced diabetic mice had increased amounts or a Hb A_{Ic}-like hemoglobin. Similar levels of this minor Hb was also found in chemically induced diabetic mice.

Numerous studies conducted since then (cited earlier) strongly suggested that increased glycosylated Hb levels in diabetic subjects are an acquired problem due to impairment of carbohydrate metabolism. In addition, patients having diabetes secondary to Cushing's syndrome had elevated glycosylated hemoglobin levels indistinguishable from idiopathic diabetes mellitus (24). Randomly determined Hb A_I or Hb A_{Ic} levels have been found to correlate to a variable degree with random blood glucose, fasting blood glucose, mean daily blood glucose during the preceding 3 months, maximum glucose concentration in the area under an oral glucose tolerance test curve, the sum of bracketed blood glucose values around meals, the highest mean glucose level during 12 hr of continuous glucose monitoring, and 24-hr urine glucose obtained 4-12 weeks previously (7,9,13,15,25). In addition, other metabolic parameters, such as serum cholesterol and triglyceride levels, have been correlated with glycosylated hemoglobin levels. If glycosylated hemoglobin is an indicator of the degree of metabolic control of diabetes, varying degrees of control and extents of hyperglycemia are expected to correlate with glycosylated levels. Using a variety of techniques to determine glycosylated hemoglobin and various approaches to assess metabolic control of diabetes, this has been well documented. (This aspect has been discussed earlier in this section.) Another way to find out if glycosylated hemoglobin level is influenced by metabolic events is by studying the effect of symptomatic hypoglycemia on glycosylated hemoglobin levels. Interestingly, diabetic patients' Hb A_{Ic} levels were significantly lower in patients who reported hypoglycemic reactions than in patients who did not report reactions (18) (Fig. 5.8).

C. Detection of Diabetes

Hemoglobin A_{Ic} has been proposed as an integrator of mean plasma glucose concentrations during the 2 months before measurement. Thus, it serves as a tool to evaluate long-term plasma glucose control in diabetics. It has been proposed by some investigators that Hb A_{Ic} measurement may also serve as a sensitive and convenient marker for the diagnosis of diabetes and thus replace the oral glucose tolerance test (OGTT) (26,27). According to Dunn et al. (27), Hb A_{Ic} is highly reproducible and responsive to minor degrees of abnormality of glucose tolerance and may provide an alternative method for defining carbohydrate tolerance or the degree of blood sugar control. The mean Hb A_{Ic} in 165 carbohydrate-tolerant subjects was 4.97 ± 0.50% (4.0-6.0%), whereas in 63 carbohydrate-intolerant subjects, this value (6.45 ± 1.14%) was significantly greater. In both groups, Hb A_{Ic} correlated significantly with the fasting blood glucose but not with the glucose tolerance test. Highly significant relationship between Hb A_{Ic} and both the fasting and 2-hr postprandial plasma glucose levels were reported by Goldstein et al. (18).

Studies conducted in a number of other laboratories failed to establish a clear-cut relationship between Hb A_{Ic} levels and the results of OGTT. In a study of 63 subjects preselected because of postprandial hyperglycemia, Hb A_{Ic} levels were compared to the plasma glucose responses at 1 and 2 hr of an oral glucose tolerance test (28). The OGTT responses were diabeticlike in 21, indeterminate in 14, and normal in 27 subjects. Hemoglobin A_{Ic} values were within normal limits in all subjects who had a normal or indeterminate OGTT response and in 10 of 21 with a diabetic OGTT. Only about half of the patients diagnosed as having mild or chemical diabetes by OGTT had elevated Hb A_{Ic}, and an elevated Hb A_{Ic} was usually associated with 2-hr OGTT levels above 228 mg/dl. Dods and Bolmey (29) compared the oral glucose tolerance test as evaluated by six commonly used scoring methods (i.e., the Wilkerson point system, the Fajans-Conn criteria, Japan Diabetic Society, The University Group Diabetic Program, U.S. Public Health Service, and Unger evaluation method) and by Hb A_I assay for detection of diabetes. Depending on the evaluation method used for OGTT, 16.7-64.3% of those subjects diagnosed as diabetic or borderline were diagnosed normal by Hb A_I analysis. In 1981, Lev-Ran (30) reported similar observations. In 140 persons with a normal glucose tolerance test, the median Hb A_I level was 8.1% (6.5-9.0%). The Hb A_I level was not significantly different in 30 patients with impaired GTT. In all 14 patients with diabetic GTT and fasting plasma glucose level above 140 mg/dl, the Hb A_I level was above 10%. Of 25 patients with diabetic GTT but without fasting hyperglycemia, only two had Hb A_I above 10%. In the same study, the Hb A_I level correlated with the mean daily plasma glucose level in 176 insulin-dependent and in 107 non-insulin-dependent diabetics. In an earlier study by Dix et al. (31), Hb A_I values were compared with 3-hr oral glucose tolerance tests in 60 ambulatory patients suspected of having abnormal carbohydrate metabolism. In 37 patients with normal plasma glucose concentration, the range of Hb A_I was 3.0-4.7%. Of the 21 borderline diabetics, 11 had increased Hb A_I (4.8-8.0%). The difference in tolerance test results between borderline diabetics with and without increased Hb A_I was insufficient to predict the status of glycosylated hemoglobin. Also, according to Bolli et al. (32), the traditional OGTT seemed more sensitive than the Hb A_I measurement in detecting subjects with reduced carbohydrate tolerance.

It is evident that elevations of glycosylated hemoglobin imply diabetes or impaired carbohydrate tolerance. Elevated glycosylated Hb Levels provide rather specific evidence for impaired glucose tolerance, but this assay is not sensitive enough to detect all cases of impaired glucose tolerance.

D. Diabetic Pregnancy and Maternal and Fetal Glycosylated Hemoglobins

Glycosylated Hemoglobins in Diabetic Pregnant Women

One of the major goals of a physician who cares for diabetic patients during pregnancy is to achieve strict control of glucose metabolism during gestation. This is done with the hope of improving fetal outcome. However, there is no entirely satisfactory means of monitoring the degree of diabetic control during pregnancy. In addition to home monitoring ob blood glucose levels, glycosylated hemoglobin assay is a simpler and more reliable means of achieving this goal. However, before such a program is initiated, it is necessary to understand how pregnancy affects glycosylated Hb levels in general. Levels of Hb A_{Ic} seem to be lower in pregnant diabetic women than in nonpregnant diabetic women (33,34). The lower values may actually have reflected better control of diabetes during pregnancy. This is also borne out by considerable difference in the fasting blood glucose levels in thes two groups. Interestingly, according to two groups of investigators (34,35), in a nondiabetic, normal pregnancy, a significant decrease in glycosylated hemoglobin seems to occur by about 20 weeks of gestation, and this reduced level is maintained throughout the rest of pregnancy. This conclusion, however, is controversial because there is no general agreement concerning such a decrease in glycosylated hemoglobin in normal pregnancy (33,36,37). It is possible that even normal pregnant women, who generally adhere to stricter dietary regimen, may have slightly reduced levels of glycosylated hemoglobin. Nevertheless, whether certain metabolic or hormonal changes in pregnant subjects can have a specific effect on glycosylation is not known. There are several changes women normally undergo during pregnancy that could be responsible for the decreased levels of glycosylated hemoglobin observed in diabetic or nondiabetic pregnant women. At 10 weeks of gestation, the fasting blood glucose is lower in pregnant than in nonpregnant women, and the reduced level is maintained for the rest of pregnancy (38,39). Moreover, in most nondiabetic pregnant women, their blood glucose levels return to the fasting concentration 2 hr after glucose ingestion, and, with four meals per day, the glucose level should be near the lower fasting value for about 16 hr per day. Blood volume increases throughout pregnancy because of an inflex of new young erythrocytes (40). This progressive increase in red cell mass would in effect "dilute" the total glycosylated hemoglobin.

Once the above-mentioned facts are taken into consideration, glycosylated hemoglobin can be used as an index of long-term blood glucose regulation in diabetic pregnancies (36,40-45). Despite the presence of the lower levels of Hb A_{Ic} in diabetic pregnant women than in nonpregnant diabetic women, Hb A_{Ic} concentrations accurately reflect the average serum glucose concentrations for the preceeding 60 days in the former group. O'Shaughnessay et al. (36) confirmed that glycosylated hemoglobin (Hb A_I) levels did reflect diabetes control during pregnancy and that Hb A_I levels were correlated with serial fasting blood sugar determined in samples drawn up to 16 weeks prior to the measurement of Hb A_I, although the highest correlation was with the blood glucose for the samples collected 8 weeks prior to Hb A_I determination. Fadel et al. (37) extended this work, including class A diabetic patients, and showed statistically significant elevation of Hb A_{Ic} in these patients as compared to nonpregnant and normal pregnant women. Widness et al. (46) performed a sequential study of glycosylated hemoglobins during diabetic pregnancies; Hb A_{Ic} was studied sequentially and postpartum in 53 women. In a group of nondiabetic pregnant women, Hb A_{Ic} fell significantly from the first to the third trimester and then rose to first trimester levels by 3 months postpartum. Hemoglobin A_{Ic} levels of type I diabetic pregnant women followed a similar pattern but at significantly elevated levels compared to nondiabetic women. Pregnant women with type II diabetes, however, did not show any such change of Hb A_{Ic} with time, despite the fact that they had elevated levels of Hb A_{Ic} during the third trimester and before 12 weeks postpartum. These fluctuations in Hb A_{Ic} levels have been interpreted to be due to changes in long-term blood glucose control. Correlations between glycosylated Hb level at 36 weeks and the fasting blood glucose level at 32 weeks (41), between the mean of four daily capillary blood glucose determinations and Hb A_{Ic} determined at the end of a 4-week period (42), and between fasting blood glucose and the Hb A_I value up to 16 weeks prior to the determination of Hb A_I (36) were reported. Since Hb F coelutes with the A_{Ic} in all the ion exchange chromatographic methods, and pregnant women are likely to have slightly elevated Hb F, Hb F may be quantitated separately and subtracted from Hb A_{Ic} values. Specific radioimmunoassay for Hb A_{Ic} or affinity chromatographic determination of GHb may be used as alternate approaches. In fact, by means of a specific radioimmunoassay, it was confirmed that Hb A_{Ic} concentration accurately reflects mean serum glucose concentration during pregnancy (46).

Fetal macrosomia is a characteristic feature of diabetic pregnancy and is believed to be the result of the growth promoting influence of insulin, which is secreted in excess by fetal pancreatic cells in response to fetal hyperglycemia secondary to maternal hyperglycemia (47). If this theory (Pedersen theory) is valid, the degree of macrosomia should correlate with fetal and maternal levels of blood glucose and with glycosylated hemoglobin levels. Widness and associates (45) reported that birth weight (birth weight ratio) correlates well with maternal Hb A_I levels and that one can predict the birth weight from Hb A_I value. Fadel et al. (37) did not confirm this finding and postulated that this lack of correlation was due to a long interval between the measurement of Hb A_I and delivery. O'Shaughnessy et al. (36) also differed, finding no correlation between Hb A_I concentration in the third trimester and the birth weight of the newborn.

Glycosylated Hemoglobins in the Newborn Infants of Diabetic Women

The levels of glycosylated hemoglobins are increased in diabetic pregnant women compared to normal pregnant women. Fetal macrosomia in diabetic pregnancies has been attributed to hyperinsulinemia, which occurs in response to fetal hyperglycemia that is secondary to maternal hyperglycemia. Although the Pedersen theory is commonly accepted, direct evidence is lacking because it is not possible to determine fetal blood glucose levels during pregnancy. Cord blood glycosylated hemoglobins may reflect the average levels of fetal blood glucose in the last weeks of pregnancy, so that measurement of these could be useful in this regard. Technical difficulties in measuring true levels of glycosylated hemoglobins in cord blood samples were a serious obstacle to progress. Several studies were initiated since a Bio-Rex 70 chromatographic method was developed to quantitate Hb F_{Ic} and Hb F_{Ia+b} (48-52). Even this method is not highly satisfactory because Hb F_{Ic} contains 80-90% acetylated fetal hemoglobin, with only the remaining in the glycosylated (glucosylated) form. However, the introduction of affinity chromatography has enabled the quantitation of total glycosylated hemoglobin (GHb) in cord blood samples (51-54). Chemical methods were also successfully used for estimation of the total glycosylated hemoglobins in such samples (54).

The levels of the minor Hb components F_{Ia+b} and F_{Ic} and the major hemoglobin components F_o and A_o were measured in the cord blood of infants delivered from normal as well as diabetic (both gestational and overt) women (49). The subjects under study were divided into four groups: group 1, 20 women with no historical factors suggestive of diabetes and a normal glucose screening test; group 2, 22 women who had either historical factors suggestive of diabetes mellitus and a normal glucose screening test or an abnormal glucose screening test but a normal oral glucose tolerance test; group 3, 20 women with an abnormal glucose tolerance test, i.e., White's class A diabetics; group 4, 8 women with IDDM. Statistically significant increases in the percentage of total Hb F_I and in the ratios of Hb F_{Ic}/Hb F were observed in fetuses delivered of diabetic mothers. The magnitude of the increment was not really substantial because Hb F_{Ic} is predominantly acetylated and the diabetic women had undergone adequate metabolic control. These results seem to indicate that the fetuses of the diabetic mothers are hyperglycemic in utero.

These studies were later repeated by utilizing affinity chromatographic methodology to quantitate total glycosylated hemoglobin (55). Cord blood samples at delivery of three groups of women, namely, 20 normal women, 20 White's class A diabetics, and 8 women with IDDM, were used for this study. Glycosylated hemoglobin was determined in cord blood samples (Table 5.2), and Hb A_I and GHb in maternal blood samples (Table 5.3). The percentages of GHb in cord blood samples from infants born to mothers with IDDM were significantly elevated compared to the normal group. Cord blood samples from White's class A diabetic women did not have significantly elevated levels of GHb. Paired analysis between the mothers and their own newborns revealed no correlation for GHb in the normal group, whereas marginal correlations were observed in IDDM and White's class A diabetic groups. This work confirms that glycosylated hemoglobin is significantly elevated in the newborns of insulin-dependent diabetic mothers. Since GHb levels reflect the time-averaged blood glucose concentration in the preceeding 2 to 3 months, these results may indicate that the fetuses of IDDM mothers have mean blood sugar values higher than fetuses of normal mothers. On the basis of the maternal GHb and Hb A_I levels (Table 5.3), White's class A diabetics must have been well controlled, which explains why the GHb levels of their newborns were not different from the newborns of normal mothers.

Elseweidy et al. (51) studied the effects of in vivo aging of fetal red cells and of the mother's diabetic condition on the levels of glycosylated hemoglobin in the fetus. Cord blood red cells from newborn infants of two normal women, one woman with White's class A diabetes, and one woman with IDDM were fractionated according to their density (age) by Dextran 40 density gradient centrifugation. Each fraction was analyzed for GHb by the affinity chromatographic method. As expected, all four samples showed an increase in GHb with an increase in red cell age (Fig. 5.9). Moreover, the GHb values were significantly higher in the cell fractions from the two newborns whose mothers were diabetic. The GHb level of the newborn of the White's class A diabetic women in this study was higher probably because this woman was not under strict metabolic control. Thus, it appears that both red cell age and mother's diabetic condition influence the GHb levels in the fetus.

Table 5.2 Comparison of the Percentages of GHb in Cord Blood of Normal, White's Class A Diabetic, and Insulin-Dependent Diabetic Mothers[a]

Samples	GHb (%)
Normal group (20)[b]	4.7 ± 0.7[c] (3.3-5.8)[d]
Newborns of White's Class A diabetic mothers (20)	4.4 ± 1.2 (3-7.6)
Newborns of insulin-dependent diabetic mothers (8)	(6.2 ± 0.7)[e] (4.9-6.8)

[a]Data from Elseweidy et al. (55).
[b]Number of samples analyzed.
[c]Mean ± S.D.
[d]Range.
[e]Bartlett's Test, $p < 0.005$.

Table 5.3 Percentages of GHb and Hb A_I in Maternal Blood of Normal, White's Class A Diabetic, and Insulin-Dependent Diabetic Mothers[a]

Samples	GHb (%)	Hb A_I (%)
Normal group (20)[b]	7 ± 0.6[c] (5.9-8)[d]	7.4 ± 0.9 (6.1-8.9)
White's Class A diabetic mothers (20)	6.4 ± 1.2 (4.8-8.4)	7.10 ± 0.7 (5.9-8.3)
Insulin-dependent diabetic mothers (8)	8.9 ± 0.9[e] (7.6-9.7)	8.1 ± 1.6 (5.5-9.6)

[a]Data from Elseweidy et al. (55)
[b]Number of samples analyzed.
[c]Mean ± S.D.
[d]Range.
[e]Bartlett's test, $p < 0.005$.

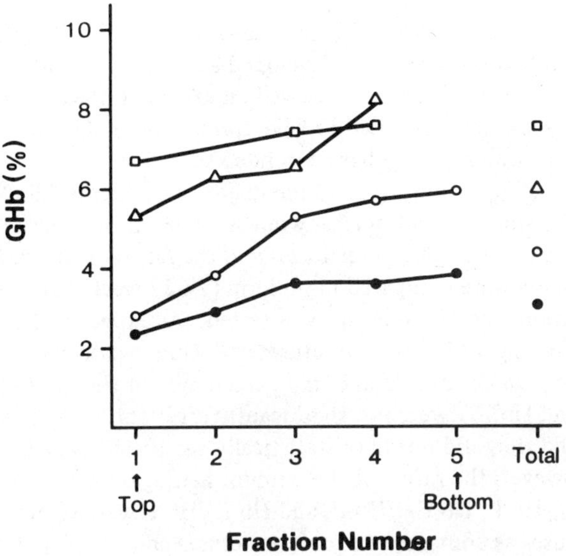

Figure 5.9 Glycosylated hemoglobin (GHb) assayed by affinity chromatography in red cell fractions isolated by Dextran 40 density gradient centrifugation from newborns of two normal women (●,○), of a woman with White's Class A diabetes (□), and of a woman with IDDM (△). From Elseweidy et al. (51) by permission of the C. V. Mosby Company.

Glycosylated Hemoglobins in the Fetus in Relation to Gestational Age

Intrauterine development correlates with changes in red cell enzymatic activity (56). Changes in red cell glycolytic enzymes might lead to changes in the levels of glycolytic intermediates, such as glucose 6-phosphate and fructose 1,6-diphosphate; these intermediates are involved in the formation of certain glycosylated minor hemoglobin components. Changes in the rate of utilization of glucose will also influence the free glucose available for glycosylation (glucosylation process). Moreover, the red cell survival time during fetal development is also expected to influence the glycosylated hemoglobin levels. For these reasons, studies have been undertaken to determine which components of cord blood hemoglobin correlate best with fetal development. Interesting relationships have emerged when the levels of the various minor hemoglobin components were correlated with gestational age. Peterson et al. (48) determined Hb A_{Ic}

by radioimmunoassay and determined Hb F_I, Hb F, and Hb A by Bio-Rex 70 chromatography in cord blood samples; they developed a clinically useful ratio of $(F_I + A_{Ic})/(F_I + A_{Ic} + A)$. This ratio showed an excellent linear correlation with gestational age and was proposed to have application in determining gestational age in the third trimester. We have extended this work by measuring the minor hemoglobins, F_{Ia+b} and F_{Ic}, and the major components, Hb A_o and Hb F_o, in cord blood samples of 44 normal women, at gestational periods ranging from 27 to 41 weeks (50). The percentages and the ratios of the various hemoglobin components were compared in preterm (27-37 weeks) and term fetuses, and their correlation to gestational age was tested. As expected, Hb F and Hb F/Hb A ratios were higher in preterm fetuses and were negatively correlated with gestational age. On the other hand, the percentages of the minor-components Hb F_{Ia+b} and Hb F_{Ic} were not significantly different in the preterm and term fetuses, and they did not have statistically significant correlation with gestational age. However, the ratios of these minor hemoglobins to the total Hb F, i.e., Hb F_{Ia+b}/Hb F, Hb F_{Ic}/Hb F, and Hb F_I/Hb F were significantly higher in term fetuses as compared to preterm fetuses and correlated positively with gestational age (Table 5.4). Thus, although the level of the total Hb F decreases as the fetus approaches maturity, relatively more Hb F undergoes posttranslational modification. The levels of the major and the minor hemoglobin components are useful for predicting gestational age with an accuracy of ±2.05 weeks. The equation describing these relationships is

$$59.46 - 0.37 \times \%\text{Hb } F_o + 0.41 \times \%\text{Hb } F_{Ic}$$

or

$$58.59 - 0.36 \times \%\text{Hb } F_o + 0.27 \times \%\text{Hb } F_I$$

Measurements of GHb, in addition to Hb F_{Ia+b} and Hb F_{Ic}, in red cell subpopulations of various ages prepared from cord blood samples of different gestational ages were also used to determine the influence of gestational age on the glycosylated hemoglobin levels in the fetus (52). Cord blood samples at gestational periods of 30-36 weeks and from a control group at 40 weeks gestational age were used in this study. Red cells of various densities (ages) were prepared by Dextran 40 density gradient centrifugation. The levels of GHb, Hb F_{Ia+b}, and Hb F_{Ic} were significantly reduced in the preterm sam-

Table 5.4 Minor and Major Hemoglobin Components in Preterm and Term Fetuses

	Preterm (N = 15)	Term (N = 29)	Significance[a] (P)
Hb F	90.8 ± 5.1	80.1 ± 7.0	0.0001
Hb A	8.4 ± 4.3	15.8 ± 5.1	0.0001
Hb F/Hb A	12.5 ± 3.9	5.6 ± 1.9	0.0001
Hb A/Hb F	0.096 ± 0.06	0.203 ± 0.08	0.0001
Hb F_{Ia+b}	4.4 ± 0.9	4.8 ± 1.3	NS[b]
Hb F_{Ic}	8.3 ± 1.0	8.5 ± 1.6	NS
Hb F_I	12.7 ± 1.5	13.3 ± 2.4	NS
$\frac{\text{Hb } F_{Ia+b}}{\text{Hb F}} \times 100$	4.9 ± 1.1	5.9 ± 1.4	0.01
$\frac{\text{Hb } F_{Ic}}{\text{Hb F}} \times 100$	9.1 ± 0.8	10.6 ± 1.5	0.0001
$\frac{\text{Hb } F_{I}}{\text{Hb F}} \times 100$	14.0 ± 1.6	16.5 ± 2.1	0.0001

[a]Student's t test.
[b]NS, not significant.
Source: From Fadel and Abraham (50) by permission of the C. V. Mosby Company.

ples compared to the term samples (Figs. 5.10 and 5.11), indicating decreased glycosylation in the preterm fetus. When the nonglycosylated hemoglobins obtained after binding the GHb to affinity gel were analyzed by Bio-Rex 70 chromatography, the acetylated form of Hb F_{Ic} also appeared to have increased with red cell age and gestational age.

Several explanations may be put forward to explain the differences in the levels of glycosylated hemoglobins between preterm and term fetuses. The rate of erythropoiesis in fetuses has been estimated to be at least three times higher than in adults (57). In fetuses, the number of reticulocytes are elevated because of an accelerated rate of erythropoiesis due to shorter red cell life span (58,59). This seems to be the reason why GHb levels in newborn infants are significantly lower than in adult life. Compared to term fetuses, higher numbers of reticulocytes are present in preterm fetuses as well, indicating a further increase in erythropoietic activity (60). Moreover, it seems that the life span of the red

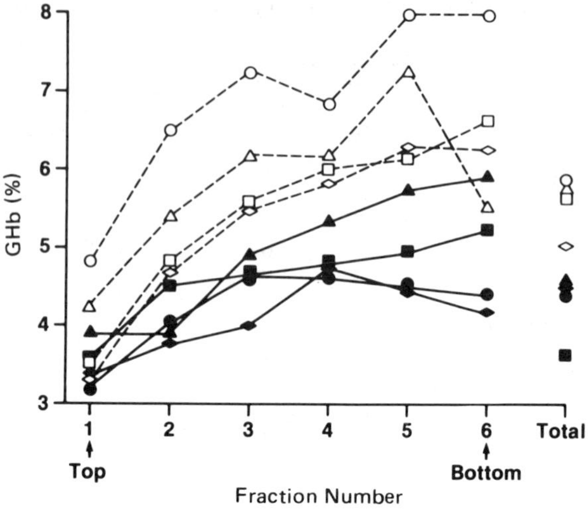

Figure 5.10 Glycosylated hemoglobin (GHb) levels determined by affinity chromatography in red cell fractions prepared by Dextran 40 density gradient centrifugation of red cells from full-term newborns (40 weeks of gestational age) (open symbols) and from those born preterm (closed symbols) at 30 (●), 31 (▲), 34 (◆), and 36 (■) weeks of gestational ages. From Elseweidy et al. (52).

cells is shorter in the preterm fetus than in the fetus at term (58,59). Thus, as the fetus matures, the life span of the red cells lengthens, gradually allowing for more exposure time of the hemoglobin molecules to glucose and glycolytic intermediates; this may explain the increased GHb in the term newborns.

E. Glycosylated Hemoglobin and the Sequelae of Diabetes

Diabetic patients from time to time suffer serious life-threatening complications due to microvascular and macrovascular changes, neuropathy, retinopathy, and nephropathy. The biochemical basis for the development for such sequelae is not known. Moreover, considerable controversy exists about the relationship of the degree of control of blood sugar to the eventual development of the sequelae. Strict control of carbohydrate metabolism should reduce the risk of secondary complications. However, it has been difficult to document this because of the lack of a means of measuring both the degree of control and the pathologic changes that occur during long-term disease. Glycosylated hemo-

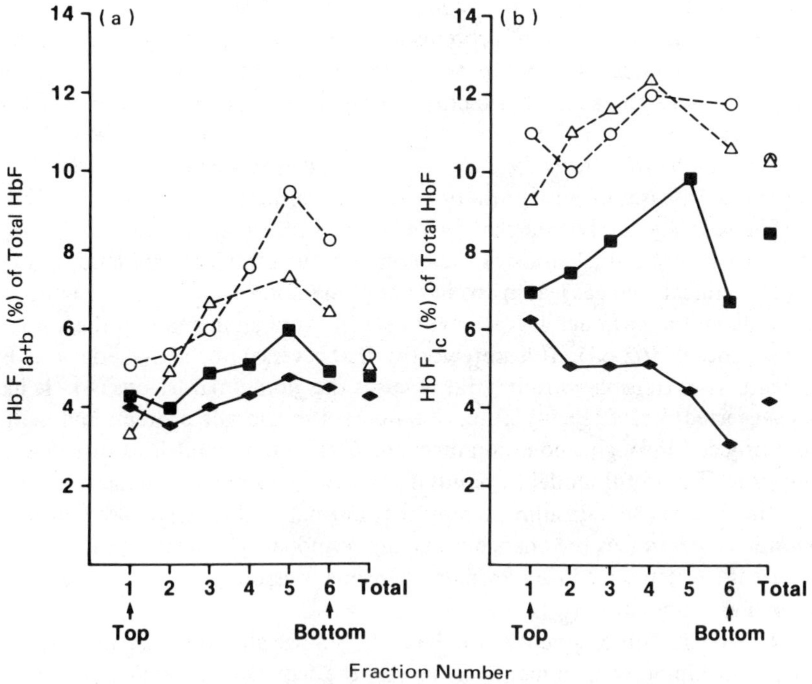

Figure 5.11 The percentages of Hb F_{Ia+b} (a) and Hb F_{Ic} (b) determined by Bio-Rex 70 chromatography in the red cell fractions of two term newborn samples of 40 weeks gestational age (○,△) and of two preterm newborn samples of 36 weeks (■) and 34 weeks (♦) gestational age. From Elseweidy et al. (52).

globin can be used as an index of metabolic control of diabetes, and glucose metabolism may be ideally controlled in this manner. In addition, glycosylated hemoglobin may provide a conceptual framework to assess the pathogenesis of the secondary sequelae of diabetes.

Some tissues in the body, red cell, lens, and nerve, for instance, do not require insulin for glucose uptake, whereas others, such as adipose or muscle, do. In the former class, the concentration of intracellular glucose merely reflects the extracellular concentration. It is noteworthy that many of the secondary complications of diabetes are manifested in tissues that are insulin independent for glucose uptake. Thus, a rise in extracellular glucose concentration that occurs in diabetes will result in a corresponding increase in the intracellular concentration of glucose and glycolytic intermediates. This leads to increased nonenzymatic glycosylation of proteins in general; hemoglobin glycosylation may serve as a model for such events. Just as glycosylation of specific sites on hemoglobin molecule alters its functional properties, glycosylation could modify enzymatic activity, half-life, solubility, etc., of other proteins as well. It may very well be that the secondary sequelae of diabetes can be considered to be due to diseases of postsynthetic protein modifications.

There is a general belief that a large number of the complications in diabetes results from a thickening of the basement membrane of capillaries (61). The biochemical changes leading to basement membrane thickening are not fully understood, although it is thought to arise from an increase in the amount of glycoproteins (62,63). It is noteworthy that reversal of the diabetic state by pancreatic islet transplantation in rat reverses the glomerular lesions (4). It has been suggested that if glycosylation of basement membrane proteins and hemoglobin proceed through a common mechanism then the monitoring of Hb A_{Ic} could provide a useful model for studying the early events of basement membrane thickening (64). Insulin therapy that normalizes blood glucose concentration in dogs reduces the chance of having retinopathy, whereas insulin therapy that is not effective in achieving euglycemia is associated with cataract formation and retinopathy (65).

Determination of glycosylated hemoglobin has allowed a reevaluation of the relationship between hyperglycemia and the sequelae. Peterson and coworkers (66) found that certain secondary sequelae of diabetes can be corrected by strict carbohydrate control, and glycosylated hemoglobin assay provides a useful means of showing the degree of control of glucose metabolism in diabetic patients. These authors emphasized the reversible hematologic sequelae of diabetes mellitus and their correlation to glycosylated hemoglobin level. White blood cell function, red cell survival, platelet hyperaggregation, and fibrinogenen survival, all improved when Hb A_{Ic} levels decreased from abnormal to nearly normal levels.

The diabetic state is associated with increased occurrence of hyperlipidemia, and abnormal lipid metabolism may be one important link between diabetes and vascular disease (67). There have been conflicting reports concerning the correlation between the glycosylated hemoglobin levels and serum lipids. A positive correlation between the concentrations of Hb A_{Ic} and serum triglycerides and cholesterol was confirmed in most studies (68-70), although no such correlation was found in some studies (71,72). The relationship between concentration of high-density lipoproteins and the control of diabetes assessed by determination of glycosylated hemoglobin was also not without ambiguity, with no correlation reported in some studies (67,70,73) and a correlation found in others (74,75). In 38 diabetic and 28 nondiabetic youths, the mean values of Hb A_I, serum cholesterol, triglycerides, and fasting plasma glucose were all significantly elevated in the diabetic group, but only Hb A_I values provided total separation of the two groups. Increased prevalence of diabetic retinopathy has been reported in patients with increased Hb A_I concentrations (21). Hormonal profiles in diabetes mellitus, including diabetic pregnancy, may vary with plasma glucose concentrations. In a study where estradiol, prolactin, and gonadotropin concentrations were measured, subnormal levels (for gestational age) were reported in type I diabetics with increased Hb A_{Ic} levels (76). By normalization of blood glucose concentrations, estradiol concentrations returned to normal range within 2 weeks and prolactin and human chorionic gonadotropin after 6 weeks, which paralleled the normalization of Hb A_{Ic} concentration. A prospective study of ten adolescent and young adult insulin-dependent diabetic patients undergoing a treatment regimen for achieving euglycemia has demonstrated improvement in microvascular and macrovascular changes while Hb A_{Ic} concentrations were lowered (26). Patients whose Hb A_{Ic} concentrations were lowered showed a decrease in basement membrane thickening. Interestingly, patients with Hb A_{Ic} concentration maintained at a higher level showed thickened capillary basement membranes. In addition, pulse volume measurements documented an improvement in blood flow to the lower extremities with a lowering of Hb A_{Ic} concentration.

F. Nonenzymatic Glycosylation and Red Cell Function in Diabetes

The organic phosphate, 2,3-DPG, is believed to play an important regulatory role in oxygen exchange by hemoglobin. As discussed earlier (Chap. 2), increased levels of 2,3-DPG lower hemoglobin oxygen affinity, thus increasing oxygen release to the tissues. Hemoglobin A_{Ic} has a high oxygen affinity, even in the presence of high concentrations of 2,3-DPG. This minor Hb will still be 50% saturated with oxygen at partial pressures where Hb A_o has already given up most of the oxygen. There is no general agreement concerning whether 2,3-DPG levels in diabetics will be different from normals. Ditzel and coworkers (77) evaluated the relationship of oxygen affinity of whole blood to red cell 2,3-DPG and Hb A_{Ic} in ambulatory nonacidotic diabetic children. Despite the fact that the diabetic children had increased hemoglobin concentration, their erythrocytes contained more 2,3-DPG than normals. This increase in 2,3-

DPG, however, did not increase the P_{50}, probably due to the presence of significant amounts of a hemoglobin, namely, Hb A_{Ic}, with high oxygen affinity. An increase in 2,3-DPG and Hb concentration compensates for the presence of a hemoglobin with high oxygen affinity (78). A separate study from the same group of investigators showed that insulin administration to diabetics with high blood glucose levels may lead to transient decreases in red cell 2,3-DPG, and in oxygen-releasing capacity of the red blood cells (79). Standl and Kolb (80) also showed no significant differences in the erythrocyte 2,3-DPG concentration between normals and diabetics. However, significant fluctuations were demonstrated during metabolic control of their diabetes. According to one study (81), blood samples from diabetics may have a P_{50} value of 24-26 mmHg as compared to 26 mmHg in normal controls. Such a small displacement in the oxygen dissociation is unlikely to have any physiological significance.

Brownlee and Cerami (1) reviewed the hematologic abnormalities in diabetic complications. Erythrocytes undergo some noteworthy changes in diabetes. Increased erythrocyte aggregation has been observed in diabetic patients, and this phenomenon appears to be more of a consequence of increased plasma protein levels than of changes in erythrocyte. This phenomenon might play an important role in the pathogenesis of microvascular sequelae. Although the abnormal red cell aggregation of diabetes does correlate with the degree of elevation of the glycosylated hemoglobin, it is not clear what role it plays in the pathogenesis of microvascular disease. Erythrocyte deformability is also significantly lowered in diabetes. Although the basis for the reduced deformability is not known, its correlation with the degree of diabetic control suggests a metabolic etiology. Miller et al. (82) showed increased nonenzymatic glycosylation of erythrocyte membrane proteins in diabetes. Peterson et al. (66) showed that diabetics have a moderately shortened erythrocyte survival. Nonenzymatic glycosylation of membrane protein may contribute to the reduced erythrocyte deformability and survival.

II. RELEVANCE OF GLYCOSYLATED HEMOGLOBINS IN HEMOLYTIC DISEASES

A. Hemolytic Anemias (Not Including Hemoglobinopathies)

Glycosylated hemoglobin levels not only depend on the blood glucose level but also on the red cell life span. A decrease in red cell survival, as in hemolytic anemia, may be reflected in a corresponding decrease in glycosylated hemoglobin levels. Horton and Huisman (83) were the first to demonstrate decreased levels of glycosylated hemoglobins in several patients with hemolytic anemia. They have determined Hb A_{Ia}, Hb A_{Ib}, and Hb A_{Ic} in patients having congenital spherocytic hemolytic anemia and autoimmune hemolytic anemia and compared these with the levels in normal controls. Hemolytic anemia was associated with devreased levels of all the three minor Hb components. Hemoglobin A_{Ia} was decreased slightly from an average of 1.0 to 0.8%, Hb A_{Ib} from 1.0 to 0.4%, and Hb A_{Ic} from 5.4 to 2.4%. The decrease in Hb A_{Ic} correlated with a rise in reticulocyte count and a decrease in blood hemoglobin level. Patients with nonhemolytic anemia, such as iron deficiency anemia and polycythemia, did not demonstrate a difference in the glycosylated hemoglobin levels. It was apparent that in the hemolytic anemia cases, Hb F, which usually elutes with Hb A_{Ic}, was slightly elevated. This means that after a correction of the Hb A_{Ic} levels for the presence of Hb F, the true Hb A_{Ic} levels in these cases would have been even lower. Bunn and his colleagues (84) confirmed this observation by determining Hb A_{Ia}, Hb A_{Ib}, and Hb A_{Ic} in five patients with hemolytic anemia and shortened red cell survival.

Panzer et al. (85) determined the glycosylated hemoglobin levels and the ^{51}Cr-labeled red cell survival in 20 patients with hemolytic anemia (14 with immune hemolytic anemia due to warm antibodies, 2 with immune hemolytic anemia due to cold antibodies, and 4 with hereditary spherocytosis), 20 patients with nonhemolytic anemia (11 patients with myeloproliferative diseases, 3 with acute lymphoblastic leukemia, 3 with iron deficiency anemia, 2 with chronic lymphoblastic leukemia, and 1 with Hodgkin's disease), and 30 healthy subjects used as controls. Significantly decreased levels of the glycosylated hemoglobin were observed in patients with hemolytic anemia (3.9 ± 0.1%), but the levels were within normal limits in patients with nonhemolytic anemia (7.0 ± 0.7%) (Fig. 5.12). When the glycosylated hemoglobin levels were correlated with ^{51}Cr-tagged red cell survival, a curvilinear correlation was found with a γ value of 0.88 ($p < 0.001$) as shown in Fig. 5.13. All patients with T_{50} RBC survival of less than 30 days had decreased levels of glycosylated hemoglobin. The level of saturation was 6.5% glycosylated Hb, which is about the mean level in two patients with hereditary spherocytosis. After successful splenectomy, glycosylated hemoglobin rose gradually within 4 weeks toward the normal range, while hematologic recovery was already complete within 1 week after operation. Thus, it appears that, as in diabetes where glycosylated Hb levels reflect the mean glucose values during the preceeding 4-8 weeks, in hemolytic anemia, glycosylated hemoglobin levels are representative of the degree of hemolysis within the preceding weeks. Determination of glycosylated hemoglobin may be useful

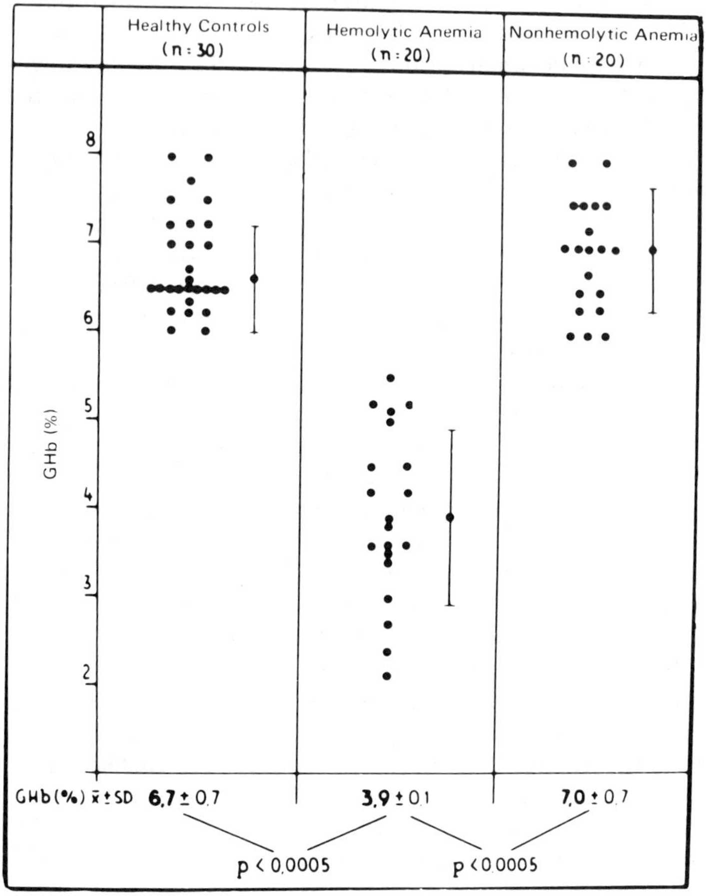

Figure 5.12 Concentration of glycosylated hemoglobin determined by a commercially available cation exchange microcolumn method in healthy controls compared to patients with hemolytic anemia and nonhemolytic anemia. From Panzer et al. (85) by permission of the author and of Grune and Stratton, Inc.

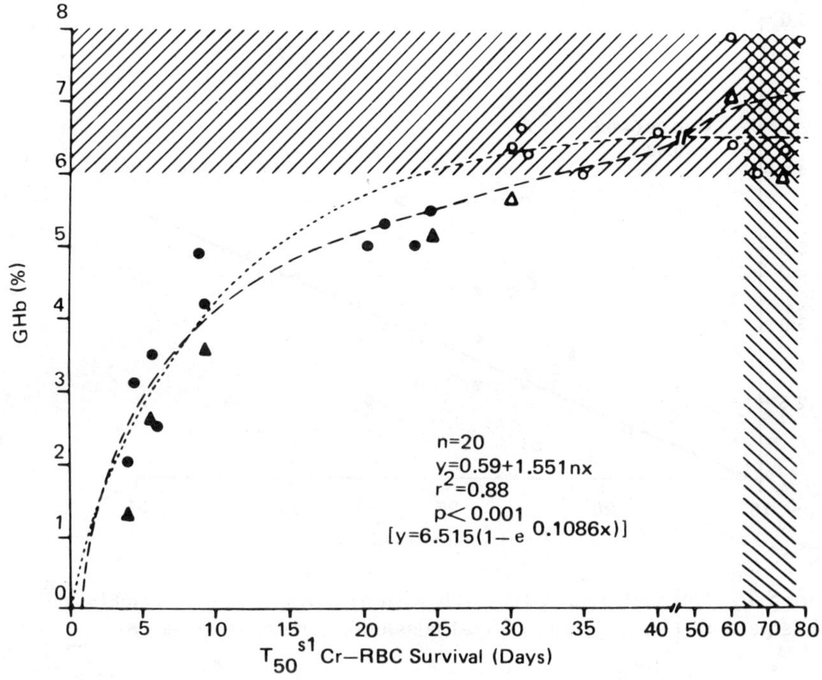

Figure 5.13 Correlation between ^{51}Cr-tagged red cell survival and glycosylated hemoglobin levels in patients with anemia. Open symbols represent patients with nonhemolytic anemia (n=10); closed symbols represent patients with hemolytic anemia (n=10); triangular symbols correspond to stable (dialyzed) glycosylated Hb levels. The broken line shows the linear regression with logarithmic abscissa; the dotted line the monoexponential model (equation in parenthesis); the hatched area indicates the normal range. From Panzer et al. (85) by permission of the author and of Grune and Stratton, Inc.

as a screening test for hemolytic anemia and for evaluation of the degree of hemolysis.

B. Hemoglobinopathies

Sickle cell disease refers collectively to a group of hematologic disorders that include homozygous sickle cell anemia (SS), S-β^+-thalassemia, S-β°-thalassemia,

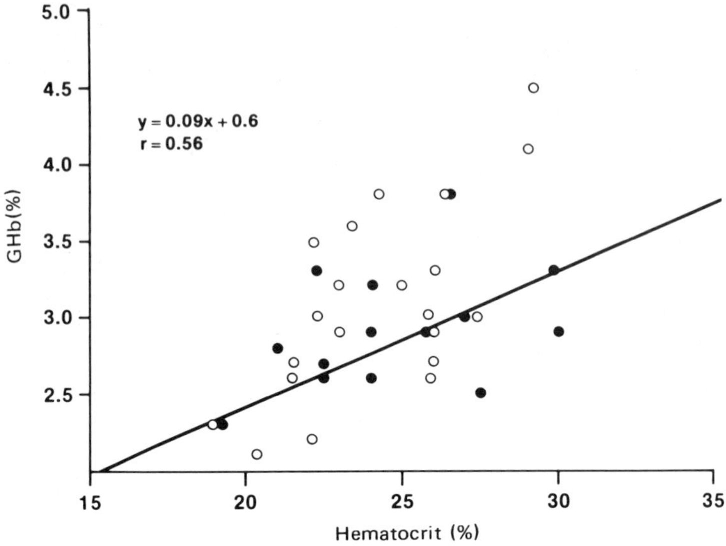

Figure 5.14 Correlation of GHb levels with hematocrit values in sickle cell anemia patients (SS) (○) and in SS-α-thalassemia-2 heterozygotes (●).

SS-α-thalassemia, SC disease, and CC condition (Chap. 2) (86). Variable degrees of hemolysis occur in these patients, and their clinical and hematological findings may reflect the extent and the frequency of such hemolytic episodes. Increased hemolysis should lead to increased reticulocyte count and decreased hemoglobin level. Sickling disorders are also generally associated with a wide range of elevated levels of fetal hemoglobin. Red cells that contain predominantly Hb F seem to have a longer survival time than cells that contain mainly sickle hemoglobin (86,87). For these reasons, Elseweidy and Abraham (88) have attempted to correlate the levels of GHb with the Hb F levels and with various hematologic parameters in SS, SC, CC, S-β°-thalassemia, and S-β^{+}-thalassemia patients. The glycosylated hemoglobin (GHb) levels were determined by affinity chromatography, and Hb S_I and Hb F by conventional Bio-Rex 70 chromatography. As expected, a positive correlation (γ=0.58) of the hematocrit values (Fig. 5.14) and a negative correlation (γ-0.55) of the reticulocyte counts (Fig. 5.15) with the GHb levels were noticed in these patients. When the GHb levels in the SS patients were compared with Hb F levels, a strong positive correlation was seen with a γ value of 0.81 (Fig. 5.16).

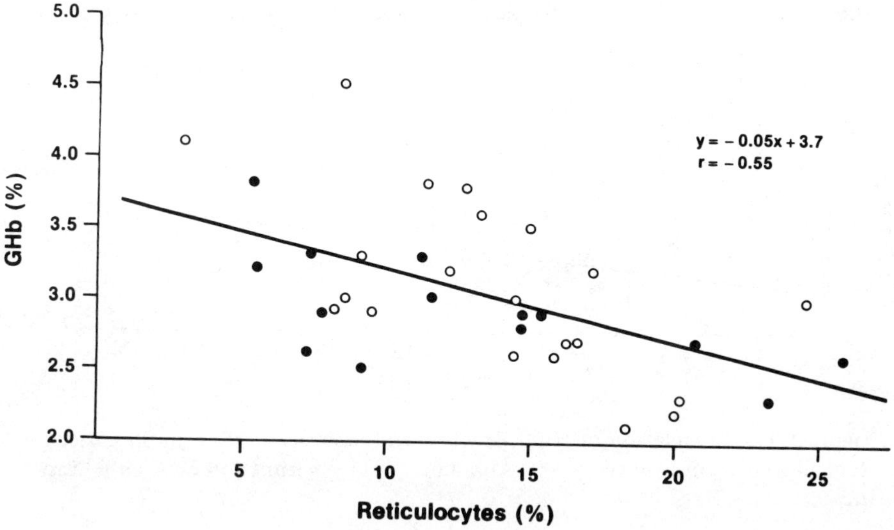

Figure 5.15 Correlation of GHb levels with reticulocyte counts in sickle cell anemia patients (SS) (○) and in SS-β-thalassemia-2 heterozygotes (●).

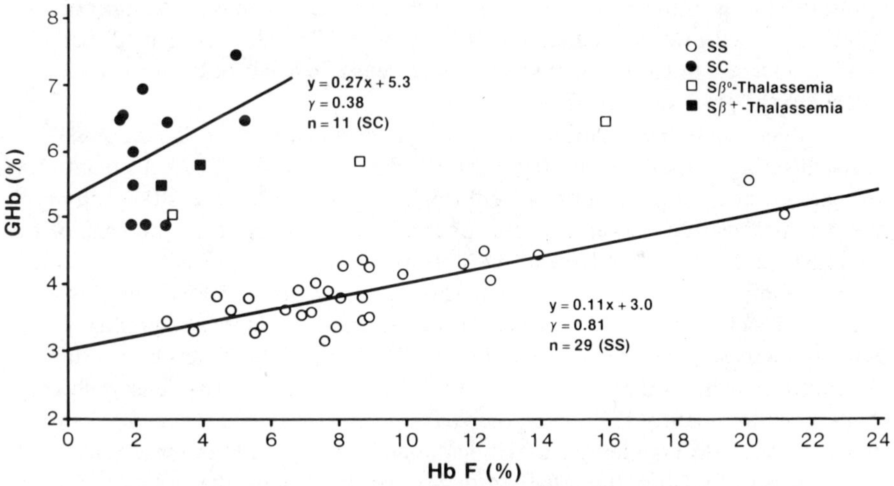

Figure 5.16 Correlation of GHb levels with the levels of Hb F in SS (○), SC (●), S-β°-thalassemia (□), and in S-β^{+}-thalassemia (■) patients. Reproduced from Elseweidy and Abraham (88) by permission of Alan R. Liss, Inc.

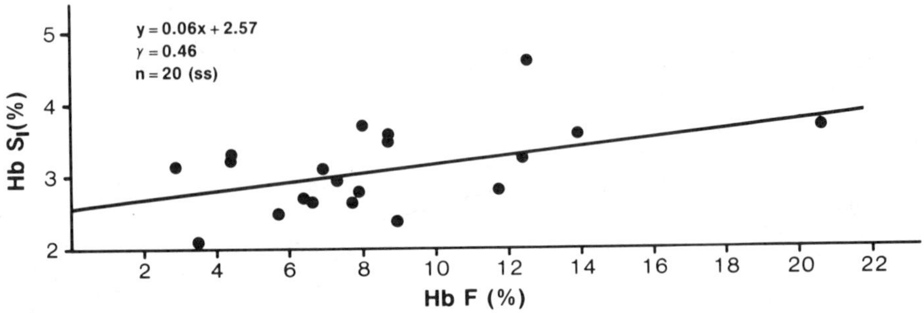

Figure 5.17 Correlation of Hb S_I levels with the levels of Hb F in SS patients. Reproduced from Elseweidy and Abraham (88) by permission of Alan R. Liss, Inc.

A similar but rather moderate (γ=0.38) relationship was seen in the SC patients. Even with three patients, a strong correlation was apparent in the S-β^o-thalassemia patients. Thus, within each group of patients (SS, SC, etc.), but not among the various groups, there existed a direct correlation of the GHb levels with the levels of Hb F. In the SS patients, there was also a reasonable correlation of Hb F values with the percentages of Hb S_I (Fig. 5.17). Thus, it seemed that with an increase in Hb F, there was an increase in the levels of both the total GHb and the glycosylated Hb S.

Glycosylated hemoglobin levels were determined in red cell subpopulations differing in their density (age) and Hb F content (88). Red cells from three SS patients and a normal control were fractionated with Dextran 40 density gradient centrifugation. Seven discrete zones of red cells were seen with each of the sample (Fig. 5.18). The fifth and the sixth zones (from the top) were combined. The bottom fractions from the SS patients contained about 80% irreversibly sickled cells (ISC's). The GHb levels in the cell fractions increased gradually with an increase in red cell density (Fig. 5.19). Hemoglobin F levels also showed a parallel increase in these cell fractions (Fig. 5.19). In the most dense cells containing predominantly ISCs, both the GHb and the Hb F values decreased sharply. The cells with high levels of GHb had high levels of Hb F and vice versa. Lower levels of GHb in the ISC fraction are consistent with the concept that these cells are indeed relatively young cells (87).

There can be at least three mechanisms by which Hb F may be influencing the levels of GHb: (a) This effect may be due to a preferential glycosylation of Hb F_o. However, the results of in vitro glycosylation studies (89) and the

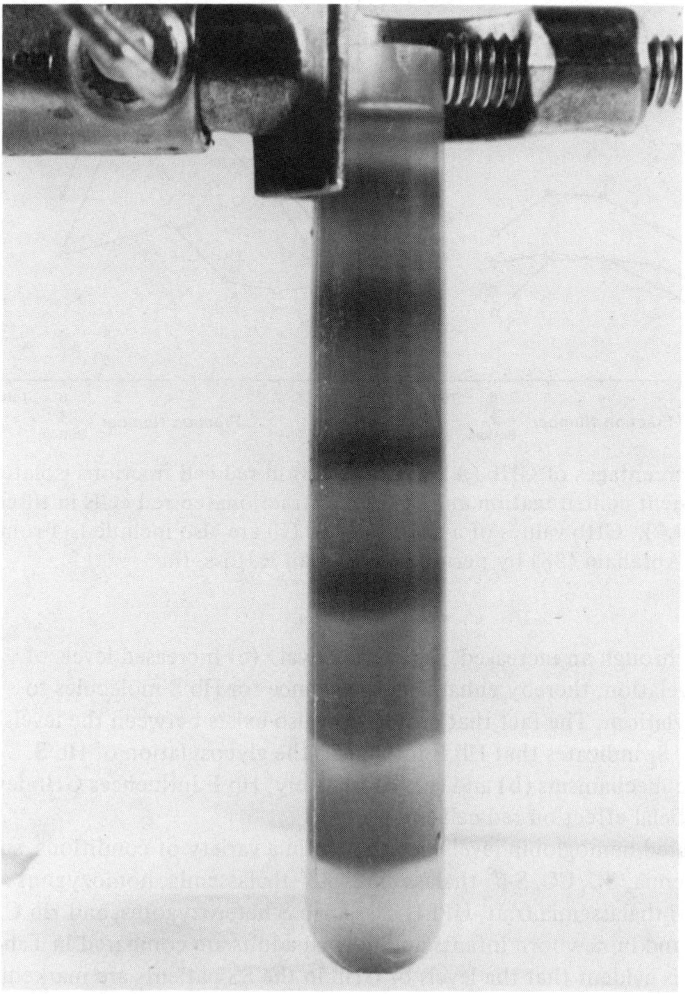

Figure 5.18 Dextran 40 discontinuous density gradient separation of red cells in a sickle cell anemia patient; see Fig. 3.7 for further details.

presence of normal levels of GHb in a homozygote for hereditary persistence of fetal hemoglobin (53) and slightly less than normal levels of GHb in newborn infants (53,54,55) does not support this. (b) Increased levels of Hb F influence

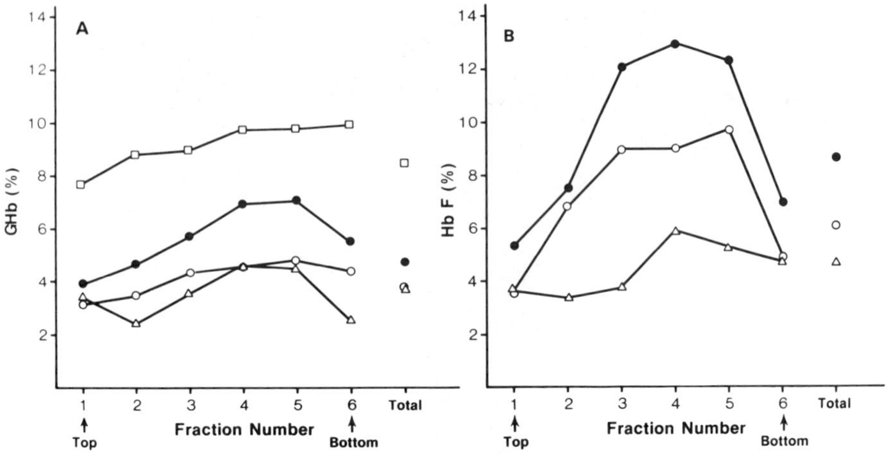

Figure 5.19 Percentages of GHb (A) and Hb F (B) in red cell fractions isolated by density gradient centrifugation and in total unfractionated red cells in three SS patients (○,●,△). GHb values of a normal adult (□) are also included. From Elseweidy and Abraham (88) by permission of Alan R. Liss, Inc.

the GHb levels through an increased, red cell survival. (c) Increased levels of Hb F decrease gelation, thereby enhancing the chance for Hb S molecules to undergo glycosylation. The fact that correlation also exists between the levels of Hb F and Hb S_I indicates that Hb F influences the glycosylation of Hb S, probably by the mechanisms (b) and (c). Most likely, Hb F influences GHb levels through a beneficial effect on red cell survival.

Glycosylated hemoglobin levels determined in a variety of conditions, such as sickle cell anemia, SC, CC, S-β°-thalassemia, S-β^{+}-thalassemia, homozygous β^{+}-thalassemia, β-thalassemia trait, HPFH cases, Hb S heterozygotes, and Hb C heterozygotes, and in newborn infants and normal adults are compared in Table 5.5 (53,88). It is evident that the levels of GHb in the SS patients are markedly lower than in the normal or in the sickle trait persons. This merely reflects the fact that the SS patients have varying degrees of hemolytic anemia. It is noteworthy that SC, S-β^{+}-thalassemia, and S-β°-thalassemia patients have normal levels of GHb. It should be pointed out that it has been well established that these conditions are associated with a much milder course of the disease than sickle cell anemia (87). The CC patients have slightly higher GHb values than SS patients, but significantly lower than normals. On the contrary, Hb C traits

Table 5.5 Levels of GHb in Various Hemoglobinopathies

	GHb (%)	
	Mean ± S.D.	Range
Sickle Cell Anemia (29)[a]	3.9 ± 0.6	3.3-4.7
SC Disease (11)	6.0 ± 0.9	5.3-7.4
S-β^{o}-Thalassemia (3)	5.6 ± 0.4	5.1-6.0
S-β^{+}-Thalassemia (2)	5.7	-
Homozygous β^{+}-Thalassemia (1)	4.2	-
CC Disease (4)	4.6 ± 0.5	4.0-5.3
HPFH Homozygote (1)	5.2	-
Hb S Trait (16)	6.7 ± 0.9	5.2-7.7
Hb C trait (18)	5.3 ± 0.5	4.4-6.2
β-Thalassemia Trait (3)	5.1 ± 0.4	4.6-5.6
Newborn Infants (30)	4.6 ± 0.8	3.3-5.7
Normal Adults (40)	6.6 ± 0.7	5.0-7.6

[a]Number of samples analyzed.
Source: From Abraham et al. (53) and Elseweidy and Abraham (88).

have GHb values lower than in Hb S traits. One homozygous β^{+}-thalassemia patient has below normal level of GHb in contrast to the β-thalassemia trait subjects having normal levels. One heterozygote for HPFH (35% Hb F) with uncontrolled IDDM has 20% GHb. A nondiabetic HPFH homozygote (100% Hb F), however, has only 5.2% GHb. A direct correlation of glycosylated hemoglobin levels with red cell life span has yet to be established in patients with sickle cell anemia and related conditions. However, the correlation of GHb levels with the levels of Hb F, hematocrit, and reticulocytes and the presence of normal levels of GHb in SC and S-β-thalassemia patients with less severe hemolytic anemia seem to indicate that determination of glycosylated hemoglobin may have an application in the evaluation of patients with sickle cell disease.

In earlier chapters (Chaps. 3 and 4), quantitative data concerning the glycosylated minor hemoglobin components in some hemoglobinopathies were presented. The separation and quantitation of the various minor hemoglobins were achieved by either Bio-Rex 70 macrochromatography or HPLC.

Several of the samples included in this study came from diabetic patients who also were either homozygous or heterozygous for Hb S or Hb C. Decreased levels of glycosylated hemoglobins were observed in nondiabetic sickle cell anemia patients. One 20-year-old Black female with sickle cell anemia and uncontrolled type I diabetes had about 16% Hb S_{Ic} and 3% Hb S_{Ia+b} (total 19% Hb S_I) (90). The quantity of this minor Hb was extremely high for a diabetic patient who had hemolytic anemia. It is not clear whether this reflects a faster glycosylation of Hb S in vivo in diabetic patients. When hemolytic anemia and diabetic condition coexist, as in this example, the interpretation of the result is rather difficult. Hemolytic anemia tends to lower and diabetes tends to raise the glycosylated Hb levels.

C. Effect of Glycosylation on Oxygenation, Gelation, and Sickling

There are numerous examples of chemical modifications of specific amino acid residues on the β polypeptide chains that increase the oxygen affinity of hemoglobin S and lead to prevention of gelation and sickling (89). Several of the aldehyde compounds, such as glyceraldehyde and pyridoxal sulfate, form Schiff-base adducts with Hb S and inhibit gelation but do not affect oxygen affinity. Glycosylation of hemoglobin A involves, in addition to the β-chain and the α-chain amino-terminal amino acids, several lysine residues on both the chains (91,92). These are α-Lys-16, α-Lys-7, β-Lys-66, β-Lys-17, and β-Lys-120. The same sites seem to be glycosylated in Hb S as well. It has been shown that certain lysine residues that can be glycosylated (β-Lys-66 and α-Lys-16) are also known to participate directly in intermolecular contacts that are important in the gelation of Hb S, and the other lysines, which are susceptible to glycosylation reaction, are situated near some critical sites of contact. Thus, it is logical to assume that modification of these sites by glycosylation may disrupt these contacts and thus inhibit gelation.

Preliminary studies indicated that glycosylation of the β-chain smino terminus or the lysyl amino acids increases the solubility of Hb S (M. M. Elseweidy et al., unpublished information). The glycosylated and the nonglycosylated fractions were isolated by preparative affinity chromatography from pooled red cell hemolysates of sickle cell anemia patients. Hemoglobin S_{Ic} and glycosylated Hb S_o from the glycosylated fraction and Hb S_o from the nonglycosylated fraction were separated by Bio-Rex 70 chromatography. Hemoglobin S_{Ic} and Hb S_o constituted about 33 and 41%, respectively, of the total hemoglobin in the glycosylated fraction. The solubility of the isolated hemoglobin fractions as determined in 2.2-2.8 M phosphate increased in the following order: Hb S_o (nonglycosylated fraction), SS lysate (nonglycosylated fraction), unfractionated SS lysate, Hb S_o (glycosylated fraction), SS lysate (glycosylated fraction), and Hb S_{Ic}. Thus, it is apparent that glycosylation influences the solubility of Hb S and that it may influence gelation as well.

Hemoglobin glycosylation with glucose (glucosylation) may not have any practical antisickling application because of the slowness of the glycosylation process, requiring relatively high concentration of glucose to achieve appreciable Hb S modification. However, certain other sugars or sugar analogues that may readily modify specific lysyl amino acid residues may have application in this respect (93). For instance, when ribose was incubated with red cells from SS patients or with purified Hb S_o, it reacted with hemoglobin five- to tenfold faster than glucose. When 5, 10, 20, 50, and 100 mM ribose were incubated with red cells for 3 hr, 1.6, 3.5, 6.3, 17.7, and 35.0% of modified hemoglobin, respectively, were formed as assessed by affinity chromatography. After the incubation with ribose, the hemoglobin components were also separated by HPLC. Even with 100 mM ribose, only 10% ribosyl-Hb S_{Ic} was formed, which indicated that more than 60% of the modification took place at sites other than the β-chain amino-terminal sites. The absence of any appreciable effect on oxygen affinity supported this conclusion. It seems that ribosylation, rather than glycosylation, may find application in antisickling. However, these studies are too preliminary to allow far-reaching conclusions.

LIST OF ABBREVIATIONS

MCHC	mean cell hemoglobin concentration
NIDOM	noninsulin-dependent diabetes mellitus
OGTT	oral glucose tolerance test
TCA	trichloroacetic acid

REFERENCES

1. M. Brownlee and A. Cerami, *Ann. Rev. Biochem., 50:* 385 (1981).
2. N. H. White, S. R. Waltman, T. Krupin, and J. V. Santiago, *Diabetes, 31:* 80 (1982).
3. R. Engerman and J. M. B. Bloodworth, Jr., *Diabetes, 26:* 760 (1977).
4. S. M. Mauer, M. W. Steffers, and D. E. R. Sutherland, *Diabetes, 24:* 280 (1975).

5. G. C. Veberti, J. C. Pickup, R. J. Jarett, and H. Keen, *N. Engl. J. Med., 300:* 638 (1979).
6. G. F. Gahill, Jr., D. D. Etzwiler, and N. Freinkel, *N. Engl. J. Med., 294:* 1004 (1976).
7. R. J. Koenig, B. S. Charles, M. Peterson, R. L. Jones, C. Saudek, M. Lehrman, and A. Cerami, *N. Engl. J. Med., 295,* 417 (1976).
8. C. M. Peterson, R. L. Jones, A. Dupuis, B. S. Levine, R. Bernstein, and M. O'Shea, *Diabetes Care, 2:* 329 (1979).
9. B. Gonen, A. H. Rubenstein, H. Rochman, S. P. Tanega, and D. L. Horwitz, *Lancet, 2:* 734 (1977).
10. E. C. Abraham, T. A. Huff, N. D. Cope, J. B. Wilson, Jr., E. D. Bransome, Jr., and T. H. J. Huisman, *Diabetes, 27:* 931 (1978).
11. M. H. Blanc, D. M. Barnett, R. E. Gleason, P. J. Dunn, and J. S. Soeldner, *Diabetes Care, 4:* 349 (1981).
12. R. E. Davis, D. J. Nicol, V. J. McCann, and J. S. Calder, *Med. J. Aust., 1:* 530 (1978).
13. J. Ditzel and J. J. Kjaergaard, *Br. Med. J., 1:* 741 (1978).
14. R. L. Jackson, R. L. Hess, and J. D. England, *Diabetes Care, 2:* 391 (1979).
15. K. H. Gabbay, K. Hasty, J. L. Breslow, R. C. Ellison, H. F. Bunn, and P. M. Gallop, *J. Clin. Endocrinol. Metab., 44:* 859 (1977).
16. P. J. Dunn, R. A. Cole, J. S. Soeldner, R. E. Gleason, E. Kwa, H. Firoozabadi, D. Younger, and C. A. Graham, *Diabetologia, 17:* 213 (1979).
17. P. J. Dunn, R. A. Cole, J. S. Soeldner, and R. E. Gleason, *J. Clin. Endocrinol. Metab., 52:* 1019 (1981).
18. D. E. Goldstein, K. M. Parker, J. D. England, J. E. England, Jr., H. M. Wiedmeyer, S. S. Rawlings, R. Hess, R. R. Little, J. F. Simonds, and R. P. Breyfogle, *Diabetes, 31* (Suppl. 3): 70 (1982).
19. B. F. Clarke, in: *The Role of Sulfonyl Ureas in the Treatment of Insulin-Independent Diabetes,* New York: *Science and Medicine,* pp. 18-23 (1980).
20. G. Boden, R. W. Master, and S. S. Gorden, *Ann. Intern. Med., 92:* 357 (1980).
21. J. Chou, C. A. Robinson, Jr., and A. L. Siegel, *Clin. Chem., 24:* 1708 (1978).
22. E. V. Flock, P. H. Bennett, and P. J. Savage, *Diabetes, 28:* 984 (1979).
23. R. B. Tattersal, D. A. Pyke, H. M. Ranney, and S. M. Bruckheimer, *N. Engl. J. Med., 293:* 1171 (1975).
24. M. D. Siperstein, D. W. Foster, H. C. Knowles, Jr., R. Levine, L. L. Madison, and J. Roth, *N. Engl. J. Med., 296:* 1060 (1977).
25. S. G. Welch and B. J. Boucher, *Diabetologia, 14:* 209 (1978).
26. L. Jovanovic and C. E. Peterson, *Am. J. Med., 70:* 331 (1981).
27. P. J. Dunn, R. A. Cole, J. S. Soeldner, and R. E. Gleason, *Ann. Int. Med., 91:* 390 (1979).

28. J. V. Santiago, J. E. Davis, and F. Fisher, *J. Clin. Endocrinol. Metab., 47:* 578 (1978).
29. R. F. Dods and C. Bolmey, *Clin. Chem., 25:* 764 (1979).
30. A. Lev-Ran, *Arch. Int. Med., 141:* 747 (1981).
31. D. Dix, P. Cohen, S. Kingsley, J. Senkbell, and K. Sexton, *Clin. Chem., 25:* 877 (1979).
32. G. Bolli, P. Compagnucci, M. G. Cartechine, F Santeusanio, C. Cirotto, L. Scionti, and P. Brunetti, *Diabetes, 29:* 272 (1980).
33. H. C. Schwartz, K. C. King, A. L. Schwartz, D. Edmunds, and R. Schwartz, *Diabetes, 25:* 1118 (1976).
34. E. P. Paulsen and M. Koury, *Diabetes, 25:* 890 (1976).
35. J. A. Widness, H. C. Schwartz, and D. Thompson, *J. Pediatr., 92:* 8 (1978).
36. R. O'Shaughnessy, J. Russ, and F. P. Zuspan, *Am. J. Obstet. Gynecol., 135:* 783 (1979).
37. H. E. Fadel, S. D. Hammond, T. A. Huff, and R. J. Harp, *Obstet. Gynecol., 54:* 322 (1979).
38. J. E. Tyson and R. A. Hock, *Am. J. Obstet. Gynecol., 125:* 1009 (1976).
39. T. Lind, W. Z. Billewicz, and G. Brown, *J. Obstet. Gynecol. Br. Common., 80:* 1033 (1973).
40. J. A. Pritchard and R. H. Adams, *Am. J. Obstet. Gynecol., 79:* 750 (1960).
41. R. D. G. Leslie, D. A. Pyke, P. N. John, and J. M. White, *Lancet, 2:* 958 (1978).
42. J. M. Miller, M. C. Crenshaw, and S. I. Welt, *J. Am. Med. Assoc., 242:* 2785 (1979).
43. J. J. Kaergaard and J. Ditzel, *Diabetes, 28:* 694 (1979).
44. A. M. Vintzileos and J. P. Thompson, *Obstet. Gynecol., 56:* 435 (1980).
45. J. A. Widness, H. C. Schwartz, D. Thompson, C. B. Kahn, W. Oh, and R. Schwartz, *Br. J. Obstet. Gynecol., 85:* 812 (1978).
46. J. A. Widness, H. C. Schwartz, C. B. Kahn, W. Oh, and R. Schwartz, *Am. J. Obstet. Gynecol., 136:* 1024 (1980).
47. J. Pedersen, *The Pregnant Diabetic and Her Newborn,* 2nd ed., pp. 211, Williams and Wilkins, Co., Baltimore, (1977).
48. C. M. Peterson, G. Kalan, L. Jovanovic, and R. Jovanovic, *Am. J. Obstet. Gynecol., 135:* 85 (1979).
49. H. E. Fadel, A. Reynolds, M. Stallings, and E. C. Abraham, *Am. J. Obstet. Gynecol., 139:* 397 (1981).
50. H. E. Fadel and E. C. Abraham, *Am. J. Obstet. Gynecol., 141:* 704 (1981).
51. M. M. Elseweidy, M. Stallings, and E. C. Abraham, *J. Lab. Clin. Med., 102:* 628 (1983).
52. M. M. Elseweidy, H. E. Fadel, and E. C. Abraham, *Hemoglobin, 8:* 363 (1984).
53. E. C. Abraham, R. E. Perry, and M. Stallings, *J. Lab. Clin. Med., 102:* 187 (1983).

54. E. C. Abraham, M. Stallings, A. Abraham, and M. M. Elseweidy, *Hemoglobin, 7:* 449 (1983).
55. M. M. Elseweidy, H. E. Fadel, and E. C. Abraham, *Pediatr. Res., 18:* 767 (1984).
56. F. A. Oski, *Pediatrics, 44:* 84 (1969).
57. A. Zipursky, *Semin. Hematol., 2:* 167 (1965).
58. H. A. Pearson, *J. Pediatr., 70:* 166 (1967).
59. M. Gahr, H. Meves, and W. Schroter, *Pediatr. Res., 13:* 1231 (1979).
60. R. C. Nerhout and P. Sturgeon, Disorders of hematopoiesis, in: *Pathophysiology of Gestation,* (N. S. Assali and C. R. Brinkman, III, Eds.), Vol. 3, p. 335, Academic Press, New York (1972).
61. J. M. B. Bloodworth, *Diabetes, 12:* 99 (1963).
62. L. Klein, D. L. Butcher, D. Sudilovsky, R. Kikkawa, and M. Miller, *Diabetes, 24:* 1057 (1975).
63. P. J. Beisswenger and R. G. Spiro, *Diabetes, 22:* 180 (1973).
64. R. J. Koenig and A. Cerami, *Proc. Natl. Acad. Sci., USA, 72:* 387 (1975).
65. J. M. D. Bloodworth, Jr. and R. L. Engerman, *Diabetes, 22i:* 290 (1973).
66. C. M. Peterson, R. L. Jones, R. J. Koenig, E. T. Melvin, and M. L. Lehrman, *Ann. Intern. Med., 86:* 425 (1977).
67. H. A. Eder, N. L. Lasser, and H. R. Scholnick, in: *Lipid Metabolism in Diabetes Mellitus: Theory and Practice,* M. Ellenberg and H. Rifkin, Eds., p. 78, McGraw-Hill, New York (1970).
68. C. M. Peterson, R. J. Koenig, R. L. Jones, D. K. Saudek, and A. Cerami, *Diabetes, 26:* 507 (1977).
69. J. M. Sosenko, J. L. Breslow, O. S. Mieltinew, and K. H. Gabbay, *N. Engl. J. Med., 302:* 650 (1980).
70. E. A. Nikkila and P. Hormila, *Diabetes, 27:* 1078 (1978).
71. H. P. Chase and A. M. Glasgow, *Am. J. Dis. Child., 130:* 1113 (1976).
72. L. Lkujber, D. Malnar, M. Kardos, V. Jaszai, G. Soltesz, and J. Mestyan, *Eur. J. Pediatr., 132:* 289 (1979).
73. G. D. Calvert, J. J. Graham, T. Mannik, P. H. Wise, and R. A. Yeates, *Lancet, 2:* 66 (1978).
74. M. F. L. Lopes-Virella, P. G. Stone, and J. A. Calwell, *Diabetologia, 13:* 285 (1977).
75. A. L. Kennedy, T. R. J. Lappin, T. D. LaVery, D. R. Haden, J. A. Weaver, and D. A. D. Montgomery, *Br. Med. J., 2:* 1191 (1978).
76. L. Jovanovic, C. M. Peterson, B. B. Saxena, Y. Dawood, and C. D. Saudek, *Am. J. Med., 68:* 105 (1980).
77. J. Ditzel, P. Jaeger, and E. Standl, *Metabolism, 27:* 927 (1978).
78. J. Ditzel, H. Andersen, and P. N. Daugaard, *Lancet, 2:* 1034 (1973).
79. J. Ditzel, H. Andersen, and P. N. Daugaard, *Acta Pediatr. Scand., 64:* 355 (1975).
80. E. Standl and K. H. Kolb, *Diabetologia, 9:* 461 (1973).

81. G. Arturson, L. Garby, M. Robert, and B. Zaar, *Scand, J. Clin. Invest., 34:* (1974).
82. J. A. Miller, E. Gravallese, and H. F. Bunn, *J. Clin. Invest., 65:* 896 (1980).
83. B. F. Horton and T. H. J. Huisman, *Fed. Proc., 23:* 430a (1964).
84. H. F. Bunn, D. N. Haney, S. Kamin, K. H. Gabbay, and P. M. Gallop, *J. Clin. Invest., 57:* 1652 (1976).
85. S. Panzer, G. Kronik, K. Lechner, P. Bettelhemi, E. Neuman, and R. Dudczak, *Blood, 59:* 1349 (1982).
86. D. F. Weatherall and J. B. Clegg, *The Thalassemia Syndromes,* 3rd Ed., Blackwell, Oxford (1981).
87. J. J. Bertles and P. F. A. Milner, *J. Clin. Invest., 47:* 1731 (1968).
88. M. M. Elseweidy and E. C. Abraham, *Am. J. Hemat., 16:* 375 (1984).
89. I. M. Klotz, D. N. Haney, and L. C. King, *Science, 213:* 724 (1981).
90. E. C. Abraham, M. Stallings, B. F. Cameron, and T. H. J. Huisman, *Biochim. Biophys. Acta, 623:* 109 (1980).
91. H. F. Bunn, R. Shapiro, M. McManus, L. Garrick, M. J. McDonald, P. M. Gallop, and K. H. Gabbay, *J. Biol. Chem., 254:* 3892 (1979).
92. R. Shapiro, M. J. McManus, C. Zalut, and H. F. Bunn, *J. Biol. Chem., 255:* 3120 (1980).
93. E. C. Abraham, M. Stallings, A. Abraham, and G. Garbutt, *Blood, 58:* 130a (1981)

6

Nonenzymatic Glycosylation of Other Proteins: A Review

I. ALBUMIN

It is not surprising from the general nature of nonenzymatic glycosylation reaction between aldose sugars and protein amino groups that numerous proteins other than Hb are glycosylated. Such events predominantly take place in tissues where the glucose transport is insulin independent. Plasma proteins, which are simply bathed in glucose medium, undergo glycosylation. Day et al. (1,2) demonstrated for the first time that human serum proteins could be glycosylated by incubating with glucose, and they showed that glycosylation of serum proteins also occurs in vivo. They incubated human serum with D-[6-^{3}H]-glucose and showed a gradual accumulation of radioactivity in acid-precipitable material. Chromatographic separation of the major three molecular weight species of serum protein (albumin, IgG, IgM) showed radioactivity associated with each. Glycosylation of albumin in vitro followed first-order kinetics with respect to albumin and glucose concentrations and occurred primarily at lysine residues. Some glucose was incorporated into lysine 189 as evidenced by indirect experiments in which acetylsalicylate, a known acetylator of lysine 189, effected a 50% reduction of glucose incorporation. On the basis of carboxymethyl cellulose chromatographic separation of glycosylated albumin from nonglycosylated albumin, glycosylated albumin represented 6-15% of the total serum albumin in normal adults. In vivo studies demonstrated that the half-life of albumin in normal rats was unaffected by the addition of 1 mol of glucose/mol of albumin. Moreover, levels of glycosylated albumin in alloxan-induced diabetic rats were elevated fourfold 4 days after withdrawal from insulin therapy.

Guthrow et al. (3) determined glycosylated albumin by ion exchange chromatography and by a chemical method [Thiobarbituric acid (TBA) assay] and Hb A_I by a microcolumn method in 25 normal and 22 diabetic patients. The column and the chemical methods were in excellent agreement, although the chemical method seems to measure more glycosylated albumin than the chromatographic method. Both procedures showed good precision and a clear separation of normal control subjects (6-9% glycosylated albumin) from poorly controlled diabetic patients (12.8-29.7% glycosylated albumin). All patients who had elevated levels of Hv A_I also had elevated glycosylated albumin. However, several patients apparently in good control based on Hb A_I measurements were found to have increased levels of glycosylated albumin. The tests for Hb A_I and for glycosylated albumin did not show any reasonable correlation. This lack of correlation was apparently due to the fact that the Hb A_I level reflects the control over the previous 1-2 months, and glycosylated albumin reflects control over a shorter period, i.e., 1-2 weeks, in keeping with its half-life of approximately 17 days (4). The concept of glycosylated albumin measurement as an index of short-term control of diabetes was strengthened in the studies followed in other laboratories. Dolhofer and Wieland (5) showed a correlation of glycosylated albumin levels with the mean blood glucose of the preceding 4 or 5 days. In addition, a decrease of glycosylated albumin of over 50% during 20 days of insulin treatment was shown in a diabetic patient, while the levels of glycosylated hemoglobin dropped only 15% over the same period (6).

Estimation of the extent of glycosylation of total protein is a much simpler approach than assaying for glycosylated albumin that requires purification of albumin from serum proteins. McFarland et al. (7) utilized a modified TBA assay for total glycosylated plasma proteins in 20 normal subjects and 29 diabetics. The method correlated well with fasting blood sugar, percent Hb A_I, and percent glycosylated albumin and also clearly separated the normal group from the diabetic group. Elevation in glycosylated albumin was responsible for only 60-70% of the total glycosylated protein. Moreover, some diabetics who appeared to be in good control based on Hb A_I measurements and fasting serum glucose showed elevation in glycosylated serum proteins. This seems to suggest that glycosylated protein assay may be a rather sensitive indicator of glucose intolerance and hyperglycemia. Since free plasma glucose was found to interfere with the TBA assay, attempts were made to improve the technique by dialyzing the serum samples or by precipitating the proteins with TCA (8-10). Kennedy et al. (11) reported a study of 107 diabetic and 82 control subjects where glycosylated protein was determined by TBA assay after dialyzing serum samples. The mean level of protein glycosylation in the diabetic group was twice that of the normal group. However, there was considerable overlap between the upper range of the control subjects and the lower range of the diabetic population. The glycosylated serum protein levels correlated with fasting serum glucose levels and Hb A_I levels. A course of treatment aimed at achieving control in eight diabetic patients resulted in about a 37% decrease in glycosylated protein in 1 week and only an 8% fall in glycosylated hemoglobin. Thus, it is apparent that glycosylated protein assay is more useful than glycosylated Hb analysis in detecting early response to treatment.

Johnson et al. (12) developed a novel manual method for measuring serum glycosylated proteins. This method relies on the ability of ketoamines (fructosamines) to act as reducing agents in alkaline solution of nitroblue tetrazolium reaction. The measurement was linear with the volume of serum assayed. It allowed clear discrimination of normal and diabetic populations and significantly correlated with fasting blood glucose concentration. Subsequently, Baker and associates (13) have evaluated the clinical usefulness of estimation of serum fructosamine concentration as a screening test for diabetes mellitus. In subjects with proved diabetes, 88% success in the detection of diabetes was possible. Likewise, only 9% false positive diagnoses were made. Lloyd and Marples (14) have adapted the colorimetric fructosamine assay for use in a centrifugal analyzer.

Affinity chromatographic methodology utilizing *m*-aminophenylboronate immobilized on agarose (Sepharose) is a relatively simple and reliable means of determining total glycosylated serum proteins (15,16). With this method, Elseweidy et al. (16) reported glycosylated protein levels of 8.8 ± 1.6% (6.4-12.8%) and 13.4 ± 3.7% (10.0-19.1%) in nondiabetic pregnant women and pregnant women with insulin-dependent diabetes mellitus (IDDM), respectively. Similar levels were also observed in a later study of normal nonpregnant subjects and nonpregnant persons with IDDM (E. C. Abraham, T. A. Huff, A. T. Varghese, A. Abraham, and M. Stallings, unpublished).

Urbanowski et al. (17) demonstrated in vitro galactosylation of purified human serum albumin with [1-^{14}C] galactose (5 mM) by incubation for 7 days under physiologic conditions. The rate of sugar incorporation into albumin increased with increasing pH and temperature and followed first-order kinetics with regard to albumin and galactose concentrations. Comparative studies indicated that the extent of nonenzymatic galactosylation was 300 times greater than glycosylation under similar conditions. It was proposed that posttranslational modification of proteins by galactosylation may be of physiologic significance in individuals with reduced galactokinase or galactose-1-phosphate uridyltransferase activities. During subsequent studies, these investigators showed elevated levels of nonenzymatically galactosylated serum slbumin in an infant with galactosemia, a molecular disease of genetic origin that is characterized by a deficiency of galactose-1-phosphate uridyltransferase (18).

II. LIPOPROTEINS

Schleicher et al. (19) showed both in vitro and in vivo glycosylation of human low-density lipoproteins (LDL) and high-density lipoproteins (HDL). In the in vitro system, the incorporation of [^{14}C] glucose was time- and concentration dependent, and was about 25% lower for both lipoprotein classes than albumin. The extent of lipoprotein glycosylation in diabetic sera was twice that in control samples. The authors pointed out that modification of lysine residues by glycosylation might contribute to increased uptake of cholesterol and to vascular complications of diabetes.

Witztum and co-workers (20) studied the effect of nonenzymatic glycosylation of LDL on its degradation. Human LDL was glycosylated by incubation with 20-80 mM glucose with or without addition of cyanoborohydrate. Glycosylation proceeded in a linear fashion, and amino acid analysis showed the presence of glucosyllysine residues. On electrophoresis on agarose gels, glycosylated LDL moved more rapidly than normal LDL. The rate of degradation of ^{125}I-labeled glycosylated LDL by cultured human fibroblasts was significantly reduced compared with native [^{125}I] -LDL. Significant effects were seen with as low as 6-15% blockage of lysine residues; high-affinity degradation was completely lost when one-third of the lysine residues were blocked. Coupling of glucose 6-phosphate to LDL also had a similar effect. Based on the NaB^3H_4 reduction and subsequent analysis of the proteins and amino acids, the existence of nonenzymatically glycosylated LDL in human plasma was demonstrated. About 1.3% of lysine residues in normal LDL were glycosylated. Yet other evidence, which supports the in vivo presence of glycosylated LDL, is the greater electrophoretic mobility on agarose of some diabetic LDL, similar to the reference glycosylated LDL. The conclusion made in this study is that since LDL undergoes nonenzymatic glycosylation, its turnover and sites of catabolism in diabetics may vary from nondiabetics. This may have far-reaching physiologic implications. It is likely that these effects are due to specific modification of lysyl groups on LDL at the LDL receptor-binding site.

Nonenzymatic glycosylation of HDL with glucose and its effect on the clearance of HDL was also investigated by Witztum et al. (21). Incubation of purified [^{3}H] glucose with HDL led to a linear incorporation of radioactivity. Glycosylated HDL had enhanced mobility when subjected to lipoprotein electrophoresis on agarose gel. When ^{3}H-labeled, glucosylated apoHDL was analyzed by sodium dodecyl sulfate (SDS)-polyacrylamide gel electrophoresis, 60-80% of incorporated radioactivity was associated with apoA-I, 10% with apoA-II, and 5-8% with apoE. When the ^{3}H-labeled, glucosylated apoHDL was subjected to amino acid analysis, the only amino acid that decreased in content was lysine, and the only new peaks noted were those coeluted with glucosyllysine. To determine the effect of glycosylation on catabolism, equal amounts of ^{125}I-labeled, glycosylated HDL and native HDL were injected into guinea pigs. In each animal, the clearance of the glycosylated HDL was more rapid than the clearance of the native HDL. When 60% of lysines were derivatized, clearance of glycosylated HDL was 60% faster than that of the control HDL. Interestingly, when as few as 2% of lysines were glycosylated, there was still an 8% increase in the rate of clearance. Accelerated clearance of the glycosylated HDL and diminished clearance of the glycosylated LDL from plasma may be contributing to the decreased HDL-LDL ratio observed in diabetic patients.

III. ERYTHROCYTE MEMBRANE PROTEINS

Bailey et al. (22) were the first to demonstrate the presence of glucose-lysine adducts in the proteins of human red cell membrane. This was observed while searching for cross-links derived from lysine-aldehydes in human erythrocytes. The major reducible components of erythrocyte membranes were shown to be hexosyllysines. Miller et al. (23) extended this work determining the extent of glycosylation in erythrocyte membrane from nondiabetic and diabetic patients. Nonenzymatic glycosylation of proteins of the erythrocyte membrane was determined by incubating erythrocyte ghosts with [^{3}H] borohydride. The membrane proteins from

18 patients with diabetes incorporated twice as much tritium as the membrane proteins from normal erythrocytes. This indicated the presence of increased levels of ketoamine in the membrane preparations from the diabetics. Subsequent electrophoretic separation of the major proteins followed by autoradiography showed ketoamine linkages in all the protein bands. No protein band showed any preferential labeling in either normal or diabetic red cells. Three patients with hemolytic anemia showed reduced incorporation of tritium from [^{3}H] borohydride, indicating decreased glycosylation due to reduced red cell survival.

Enhanced nonenzymatic glycosylation of erythrocyte membrane proteins in diabetes may have physiologic significance. It is worth pointing out that diabetics have a moderately shortened erythrocyte survival that is corrected by institution of rigid control of diabetes (24). This decreased survival may be due to diabetic red cells being less deformable than normal red cells (25). It is not certain whether the abnormal rheology of the membrane in diabetic erythrocytes is due to posttranslational modifications, such as nonenzymatic glycosylation of membrane proteins.

IV. PERIPHERAL NERVE PROTEINS

An affinity chromatographic system that selectively retains glycosylated amino acids (26) was utilized to determine the amount of glycosylation in peripheral nerve in diabetic and control rats and dogs (27). Sciatic nerves from control and alloxan-induced diabetic rats and femoral nerves from control and diabetic dogs were homogenized and treated with NaB^3H_4. After acid hydrolysis, glycosylated amino acids were separated by affinity chromatography on columns containing *m*-aminophenylboronic acid immobilized on Bio-Gel P-6. Pooled glycosylated amino acid fractions were also subjected to conventional amino acid analysis.

In all instances, the radioactivity of the effluent fractions were determined. Reduced, hydrolyzed sciatic nerve homogenates separated on affinity chromatography system gave essentially identical chromatograms to those obtained previously (27) from reduced, hydrolyzed hemoglobin and urinary amino acids and peptides. Comparison of the amount of glycosylated amino acids in sciatic nerves from diabetic rats with the amount from normal controls showed that the mean amount in the diabetic animals was 2.8 times greater than the mean value in normal animals. Glycosylated lysine constituted the major borohydride-reducible adduct present in the glycosylated amino acid isolated by affinity chromatography.

It is not certain whether nonenzymatic glycosylation of nerve protein plays a role in the development of diabetic neuropathy. However, a strong similarity between the morphological findings of cyanate-induced neuropathy (28) and those of diabetic neuropathy suggest that glucose might undergo chemical reaction similar to that of cyanate. Cyanate, which inhibits polymerization of Hb S by carbamylation of the NH_2 termini of hemoglobin S (29), also seems to carbamylate peripheral nerve proteins. It was suggested that excessive nonenzymatic glycosylation of peripheral nerve in diabetes could involve mainly myelin proteins, axonal proteins, or various components of these proteins.

V. COLLAGEN

Collagen, the main fibrous protein of the connective tissue, is the most abundantly present protein in the human body. These insoluble fibers also account for the major portion of the organic mass of skin, bone, tendon, and blood vessels (30). The unique structural and functional properties of collagen are attributed to intra- and intermolecular cross-linking of collagen fibrils (31).

Tanzer et al. (32) identified a reduced N^{ϵ}-hexosylhydroxylysine in acid hydrolysate of NaB^3H_4-reduced, insoluble calf skin collagen. This compound was postulated to represent a new structural class of cross-link, uniting collagen and extracellular carbohydrates, and was believed to be formed by Schiff-base formation between the ϵ-amino group of hydroxylysine and the carbohydrate portion of the proteoglycans and glycoproteins of connective tissue. Schiff-base formation between free hexose and the hydrosylysines of collagen was not considered a strong possibility by which this compound was formed.

Lysine and hydroxylysine residues are known to be involved in the formation of collagen cross-links. These residues are also likely targets for nonenzymatic glycosylation, the extent of which may be increased in diabetic state. Rosenberg et al. (33) attempted to explore the relationship between hyperglycemia and vascular complications of diabetes by studying the glycosylation of arterial collagen. Aortal collagen was prepared from streptozotocin-induced diabetic and nondiabetic control rats. Collagen content in each preparation was estimated by the hydroxyproline content, and protein-bound hexoses (ketoamine-linked) by a colorimetric procedure (TBA assay). Rats with acute diabetes of 6-weeks duration showed a greater degree of arterial collagen glycosylation than normal animals. Since vascular collagen is continuously exposed to high blood glucose concentrations in the diabetic state, enhanced glycosylation of ϵ-NH_2 groups of lysine and hydroxylysine is likely to occur. In diabetes, the increased glycosylation of collagen fibrils may alter the function, structure, and turnover of collagen, probably because the glucose-linked amino acids are no longer available for cross-linking.

Cohen et al. (34) reported increased nonenzymatic glycosylation of glomerular basement membrane collagen in diabetic rat. Basement membrane was purified from glomeruli isolated from normal and streptozotocin-induced diabetic rats. After extraction of the noncollagen material, the extent of glycosylation in collagen was determined colorimetrically (TBA assay). The level of glycosylation of basement membrane collagen purified from diabetic rats was significantly greater than in nondiabetic animals. Similar results were reported in human glomerular basement membrane collagen by Uitto and co-workers (35). They showed that while the enzymatic glycosylation remained unchanged in diabetes, nonenzymatic glycosylation was significantly increased. Glomerular basement membrane serves as a size- and charge-selective filtration barrier. Modification in its electrochemical properties through glycosylation of amino groups or interference with molecular packing via ketoamine linkage of ϵ-amino groups of lysine and hydroxylysine decrease the availability of these amino acids for collagen cross-linking. Such changes could affect the charge- or size-selective nature of the filtration barrier, thus, leading to proteinuria.

Bailey and co-workers (36-38) have reported studies of the age-related changes in the reducible cross-links of several types of collagen. In all the tissues studied, there was a decrease with age in the amounts of all these intermolecular cross-links. In collagen-rich tissues, the characteristic changes due to diabetes resembled changes occurring with aging (39,40). Nonenzymatic glycosylation of insoluble human tendon collagen, a protein with little or no turnover, was determined by TBA assay in 23 subjects as a function of age and the presence or absence of diabetes (39,40). Nonenzymatic glycosylation of collagen was found to increase with age and was markedly increased in IDDM. It was concluded that glucose nonenzymatically bound to human collagen may indicate the level of long-term control of diabetes and may play a role in the alteration of collagenous tissue properties that occurs in both aging and diabetics.

VI. LENS CRYSTALLINS

The lens, like the erythrocyte, is not dependent on insulin for glucose uptake, and hence the intracellular glucose concentration reflects the extracellular milieu (41). Moreover, the lens crystallins, like collagen, have little or no turnover and thus are expected to undergo significant nonenzymatic glycosylation. Stevens et al. (42) were the first to demonstrate both in vivo and in vitro glycosylation of α, β, and γ crystallins. To establish a relationship between glycosylation and cataract formation in diabetes, they have relied on in vivo studies of lenses from alloxan-induced diabetic rats, rat lenses cultured in high glucose medium, and long-term in vitro glycosylation of lens crystallins isolated from bovine lenses. Incubations of sterile crystallins revealed that the solution remained clear for several months as long as they were stored under nitrogen with dithioerythritol. In the absence of the added reducing agent, opalescence increased gradually as monitored by the absorbance at 550 nm. This development of opalescence was greatly facilitated by the presence of 50 mM glucose 6-phosphate. Both [^{14}c]glucose and [^{14}C]glucose 6-phosphate used as tracers were found in time to become associated with acid-precipitable proteins. [^{14}C]Glucose or [^{14}C]glucose 6-phosphate radioactivity was associated with all the crystallins. Rat lenses cultured in vitro in a medium containing 30 mM glucose developed an opacity that mimicked cataract. Separation of the crystallins after reduction with NaB^3H_4 indicated that α-crystallin isolated from the cultured lenses has greater amount of radioactivity, i.e., an increased number of borohydride-reducible bonds. The increase in borohydride-reducible bonds per milligram of protein per day of culture showed a linear increase with glycosylation. A similar increase in borohydride-reducible bonds was found to be associated with the crystallins of cataractous lenses isolated from diabetic rats.

According to Spector and Roy (43), the opacification of crystallin solution, however, was not simply related to the extent of glycosylation. These authors investigated the formation of high molecular weight (HMW) aggregates in opalescent solution by gel filtration chromatography. An increase in the aggregate formation occurred in both the controls and the glucose 6-phosphate-treated samples after an initial lag period of 15 days. The reduction of the disulfide bonds induced a large decrease in the HMW species. However, this reversibility was more incomplete in the glycosylated crystallin than in the control. This incomplete reduction indicates the presence of other types of intermolecular linkages. Soon after the work of Stevens et al. (42), Pande et al. (44) published results contradicting the findings of the former group. The studies were done on a large number of human normal lenses and nondiabetic, senile cataractous lenses. Examination of glycosylation was conducted utilizing NaB^3H_4. Approximately the same number of moles of tritium (0.2 mol) were incorporated per mole of protein in normal and in senile cataractous lenses with varying degrees of opacity. Protein isolated from the diabetic lenses had only slightly higher levelsof tritium incorporation. The results suggest that nonenzymatic glycosylation does not appear to be a primary factor in cataract formation. However, it should be pointed out that these studies were done mostly on senile cataractous lenses rather than diabetic cataractous lenses, and the mechanism of diabetic cataract formation could be different from senile cataract formation.

Similar studies were done by Monnier et al. (45) in cataracts formed in both diabetic and galactosemic rats. Ten- and fivefold increases in glucose- and galactose-lysine adducts were detected in diabetic and galactosemic cataractous lenses, respectively. High molecular weight aggregates were also detected. By in vitro glycosylation of bovine crystallin proteins with glucose, Avasthi et al. (46) concluded that glucose induces aggregation of crystallins by some mechanism other than the exposure of sulfhydryl groups. Liang and Chakrabarti (47), using circular dichroism (CD), demonstrated changes in the ultraviolet (uv)-CD characteristic of aromatic amino acid residues upon glycosylation of bovine lens proteins. These results indicate that glycosylation causes a change in tertiary, but not in secondary, structure of the protein molecule.

Ansari et al. (48) separated normal, senile cataractous, and diabetic cataractous lenses into water-soluble, urea-soluble, and insoluble protein fractions. Tritium incorporation (from NaB^3H_4), protein-disulfide bonds, mixed disulfide bonds, and borohydride-reducible bonds were noticed in both ures-insoluble and -soluble protein fractions from diabetic cataractous lenses. A correlation between glycosylation and sulfhydryl oxidation in diabetic cataract formation was apparent.

The lens never shed its cells, so the cells at the center of the lens are as old as the animal itself. Thus, the proteins near the center of the lens do not turnover or turnover slowly. Such long-lived proteins have a great chance to undergo posttranslational modification. As the lens ages, a high molecular weight aggregate accumulates in the soluble fraction, which is believed to be a precursor to the disulfide-linked high molecular weight protein present in the insoluble fraction (49). There is also an increase in the amount of water-insoluble protein found in the older and cataractous lenses; however, the disulfide-linked high molecular weight species is found only in cataractous lenses. Chiou et al. (50) investigated nonenzymatic glycosylation of crystallins from calf and mature bovine lenses. Reduction with NaB^3H_4 was used to determine the extent of glycosylation. They found that the tritium incorporation and the amount of glucitol-lysine adduct detected increased with age, particularly in a HMW aggregate that accumulates with aging. Crystallin fractions from the nucleus consistently showed higher specific radioactivity than the crystallins from the cortex. This difference may be explained from the difference in the turnover of the proteins in these two compartments. Perry and Abraham (51) used HPLC on molecular sieve columns to separate the various crystallins, including the HMW protein from 2-week-old rats and 2-year-old Sprague-Dawley rats that had developed cataracts. The total glycosylated proteins and amino acids were quantitated by affinity chromatographic methods. No significant amount of HMW was found in the young lenses, whereas the HMW fraction comprised 7.1% of the total soluble lens proteins from the older lenses. Reduction with dithiothreitol significantly (but not completely) reduced the HMW fraction, indicating the pressure of disulfide-linked and other forms of aggregates. Total glycosylated lens protein was 2.0% in the young animals and 5.6% in the old animals. There was a concomitant decrease in free sulfhydryl groups in the old animals, indicating possible increased disulfide formation. Thus, it appears that an interrelationship exists among the various factors, i.e., glycosylation, disulfide formation, and ultimately formation of HMW protein.

VII. INSULIN

According to Dolhofer and Wieland (52), on incubation of crystalline bovine insulin with [^{14}C] glucose and [^{3}H] mannose, the hexoses became covalently linked to the hormone. The amount of each hexose taken up by insulin proved to be a linear function of the sugar concentration up to 220 mmol/liter. At this concentration, 3.6 ± 0.39 glucose and 5.0 ± 0.43 mannose residues, respectively, were incorporated per mole of insulin. Glycosylation of insulin diminished the hormone's effect on [1-^{14}C] glucose oxidation by adipose tissue. Also, with respect to lipogenesis, the response of adipocytes was significantly lower in the presence of the glycosylated insulin as compared to the native hormone. The antilipolytic action of insulin with isolated fat cells was significantly decreased by glycosylation. On the other hand, the mannosylated insulin exhibited unchanged stimulation of glucose oxidation and only marginal lowering of antilipolysis. The immunologic reactivity of insulin was not altered by glycosylation. Although glycosylation of insulin was demonstrated in vitro, it remains to be established whether glycosylated insulin is formed in vivo under physiologic conditions.

VIII. OSTEOCALCIN

Osteocalcin constitutes about 20% of the noncollagenous proteins in bone matrix and is the eighth most abundant protein in vertebrates. This protein remains deposited in bone for long times and can become nonenzymatically glycosylated. Cow osteocalcin was found to be 10% glycosylated, whereas calf osteocalcin was only 4-5% glycosylated (53). This estimate was based on fluorometric determination of the number of glycogroups. These results were confirmed by NaB^3H_4 reduction of osteocalcin from cow and calf. The finding was consistent with the faster turnover of younger bones.

LIST OF ABBREVIATIONS

CD circular dichroism
HDL high-density lipoproteins
HMW high molecular weight
LDL low-density lipoproteins

REFERENCES

1. J. F. Day, S. R. Thorpe, and J. W. Baynes, *J. Biol. Chem., 254:* 595 (1979).
2. J. F. Day, R. W. Thornburg, S. R. Thorpe, and J. W. Baynes, *J. Biol. Chem., 254:* 9394 (1979).
3. C. E. Guthrow, M. A. Morris, J. F. Day, S. R. Thorpe, and J. W. Baynes, *Proc. Natl. Acad. Sci., USA, 76:* 4258 (1979).
4. H. E. Schultze and J. F. Heremans, *Molecular Biology of Human Proteins,* pp. 450-517 Elsevier, New York (1966).
5. R. Dolhofer and O. H. Wieland, *FEBS Lett., 103:* 282 (1979).
6. R. Dolhofer and O. H. Wieland, *Diabetes, 29:* 417 (1980).
7. K. F. McFarland, E. W. Catalano, J. F. Day, S. F. Thorpe, and J. W. Baynes, *Diabetes, 28:* 1011 (1979).
8. K. A. Ney, K. J. Colley, and S. V. Pizzo, *Anal. Biochem., 118:* 294 (1981).
9. A. L. Kennedy, T. D. Mehl, and T. J. Merimee, *Diabetes, 29:* 413 (1982).
10. A. Ma, M. A. Naughton, and D. P. Cameron, *Clin. Chim. Acta, 115:* 111 (1981).
11. A. L. Kennedy, T. D. Mehl, and T. J. Merimee, *Diabetologia, 21:* 94 (1981).
12. R. N. Johnson, P. A. Metcalf, and J. R. Baker, *Clin. Chim. Acta, 127:* 87 (1982).

13. J. R. Baker, J. P. O'Connor, P. A. Metcalf, M. R. Lawson, and R. N. Johnson, *Br. Med. J., 287:* 863 (1983).
14. D. Lloyd and J. Marples, *Clin. Chem., 30:* 1686 (1984).
15. E. C. Abraham, R. E. Perry, and M. Stallings, *J. Lab. Clin. Med., 102:* 187 (1983).
16. M. M. Elseweidy, H. E. Fadel, and E. C. Abraham, *Ped. Res., 18:* 767 (1984).
17. J. C. Urbanowski, M. A. Cohenford, and J. A. Dain, *J. Biol. Chem., 257:* 111 (1982).
18. J. C. Urbanowski, M. A. Cohenford, H. L. Levy, J. D. Crawford, and J. A. Dain, *N. Engl. J. Med., 306:* 84 (1982).
19. E. Schleicher, T. Deufeel, and O. H. Wieland, *FEBS Lett., 129:* 1 (1981).
20. J. L. Witztum, E. M. Mahoney, M. J. Branks, M. Fisher, R. Elam, and D. Steinberg, *Diabetes, 31:* 283 (1982).
21. J. L. Witztum, M. Fisher, T. Pietro, U. P. Steinbrecker, and R. L. Elam, *Diabetes, 31:* 1029 (1982).
22. A. J. Bailey, S. P. Robins, and M. J. A. Tanner, *Biochim. Biophys. Acta, 434:* 51 (1976).
23. J. A. Miller, E. Gravallese, and H. F. Bunn, *J. Clin. Invest., 65:* 896 (1980).
24. C. M. Peterson, R. V. Koenig, R. L. Jones, E. T. Melvin, and M. L. Lehrman, *Ann. Intern. Med., 86:* 425 (1977).
25. D. E. McMillan, N. G. Utterback, and J. Lapuna, *Diabetes, 27:* 895 (1978).
26. M. Brownlee, H. Vlassara, and A. Cerami, *Diabetes, 29:* 1044 (1980).
27. H. Vlassara, M. Brownlee, and A. Cerami, *Proc. Natl. Acad. Sci., USA, 78:* 5190 (1981).
28. I. Tellez-Nagel, J. K. Korthals, H. Vlassara, and A. Cerami, *J. Neuropathol. Exp. Neurol., 43:* 351 (1977).
29. A. Cerami and J. M. Manning, *Proc. Natl. Acad. Sci., USA, 68:* 1180 (1971).
30. K. I. Kivirikko and L. Risteli, *Med. Biol. 54:* 159 (1976).
31. M. L. Tanzer, *Science, 180:* 561 (1973).
32. M. L. Tanzer, R. Fairweather, and P. M. Gallop, *Arch. Biochem. Biophys., 151:* 137 (1972).
33. H. Rosenberg, J. B. Modrak, J. M. Hassing, W. A. Al-Turk, and S. J. Stohs, *Biochem. Biophys. Res. Commun., 91:* 498 (1979).
34. M. P. Cohen, E. Urdanivia, M. Surma, and V. Yu Wu, *Biochem. Biophys. Res. Commun., 95:* 765 (1980).
35. J. Uitto, G. A. Grant, A. J. Perejda, E. Rowold, and J. E. Williamson, *Fed. Proc., 39:* 1792 (1980).
36. A. J. Bailey, C. M. Peach, and L. J. Fowler, *Biochem. J., 117:* 819 (1970).

37. A. J. Bailey and M. S. Shimokomaki, *FEBS Lett., 16:* 1971).
38. S. P. Robins and A. J. Bailey, *Biochem. Biophys. Res. Commun., 48:* 76 (1972).
39. S. L. Schnider and R. R. Kohn, *J. Clin. Invest., 66:* 1179 (1980).
40. R. R. Kohn and S. L. Schnider, *Diabetes, 31* (Suppl. 3): 47 (1982).
41. R. G. Spiro, *Diabetologia, 12:* 1 (1976).
42. V. J. Stevens, C. A. Rouzer, V. M. Monnier, and A. Cerami, *Proc. Natl. Acad. Sci., USA, 75:* 2918 (1978).
43. A. Spector and D. Roy, *Proc. Natl. Acad. Sci., USA, 75:* 3244 (1978).
44. A. Pande, W. H. Garner, and A. Spector, *Biochem. Biophys. Res. Commun., 89:* 1260 (1979).
45. V. M. Monnier, J. J. Stevens, and A. Cerami, *J. Exp. Med., 50:* 1098 (1979).
46. Y. C. Avasthi, N. H. Ansari, and S. K. Srivastava. *Red Blood Cell and Lens Metabolism,* S. K. Srivastava, Ed., Elsevier, New York (1980).
47. J. N. Liang and B. Chakrabarti, *Invest. Ophthalmol., 20* (Suppl): 129 (1981).
48. N. H. Ansari, Y. C. Awasthi, and S. K. Srivastava, *Exp. Eye Res., 31:* 9 (1980).
49. D. Ray and A. Spector, *Exp. Eye Res., 22:* 273 (1976).
50. S. H. Chiou, L. T. Chylack, Jr., W. H. Tung, and H. F. Bunn, *J. Biol. Chem., 256i:* 5176 (1981).
51. R. E. Perry and E. C. Abraham, *Fed. Proc., 43:* 1706 (1984).
52. R. Dolhofer and O. H. Wieland, *FEBS Lett., 100:* 133 (1979).
53. C. M. Gundberg and P. M. Gallop, *Fed. Proc., 43:* 1671 (1984).

Index